Successful Ageing

Successful Ageing

Ambition and Ambivalence

CLEMENS TESCH-RÖMER

Director of the German Centre of Gerontology and Adjunct Professor of Psychology at the Freie Universität Berlin, German Centre of Gerontology, Berlin, Germany

HANS-WERNER WAHL

Senior-Professor and Director, Network Ageing Research & Institute of Psychology, Heidelberg University, Heidelberg, Germany

with

SURESH I. S. RATTAN

Professor Emeritus, Department of Molecular Biology and Genetics, Aarhus University, Aarhus, Denmark

LIAT AYALON

Deputy Director, Louis and Gabi Weisfeld School of Social Work, Bar Ilan University, Ramat Gan, Israel

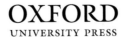

OXFORD
UNIVERSITY PRESS

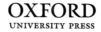

OXFORD
UNIVERSITY PRESS

Great Clarendon Street, Oxford, OX2 6DP,
United Kingdom

Oxford University Press is a department of the University of Oxford.
It furthers the University's objective of excellence in research, scholarship,
and education by publishing worldwide. Oxford is a registered trade mark of
Oxford University Press in the UK and in certain other countries

© Oxford University Press 2022

The moral rights of the authors have been asserted

First Edition published in 2022

Impression: 1

Published in the United States of America by Oxford University Press
198 Madison Avenue, New York, NY 10016, United States of America

British Library Cataloguing in Publication Data

Data available

Library of Congress Control Number: 2021940639

ISBN 978–0–19–289753–4

DOI: 10.1093/med/9780192897534.001.0001

Printed and bound by
CPI Group (UK) Ltd, Croydon, CR0 4YY

Acknowledgements

We are deeply grateful to Jamie Hyland for the excellent language editing of this text. We would also like to thank Ulrich Prachtl for the picture of the front relief of the Temple of Friendship in the palace garden of Schloss Schönbusch, Aschaffenburg, in Bavaria, Germany.

Contents

PART I

CONCEPTIONS OF SUCCESSFUL AGEING

1
History of successful ageing

A short look back into the long history of longevity and ageing

The struggle against death and the striving to live a life without end is as old as humankind itself. Ancient burial rituals, even those carried on by Neanderthals more than 100,000 years ago, whose practices included pointing graves toward the east where the sun rises, suggest a desire to help the dead continue their lives in another realm. Ancient Egyptians helped their dead to continue their existence by mummifying their bodies so that their souls would continue to have a safe dwelling place. They also symbolically reopened their mouths and reactivated their senses by ritually touching the relevant body parts to enable them to eat, speak, see, and hear. Grave chambers were also stocked with fruit and wine to give the departed's soul the sustenance it needed to 'live on' (Assmann, 2005). The *Epic of Gilgamesh* (dating to about 3000 years BCE) builds on the myth that humanity tragically lost its immortality a long time ago. There are also a great many ancient myths telling of mysterious lands somewhere on Earth where the inhabitants lead lives without death, and indeed without even growing old (Gruman, 1966).

Yet total immortality has always been looked upon as a highly ambivalent gift. The Greek legend of Tithonos illustrates both the allure and the dread of ever-lasting life. Tithonos, a prince of Troy, was the lover of Eos, the immortal goddess of the dawn. In fear of eventually losing Tithonos to death, Eos asked Zeus to make him immortal. However, she forgot to ask Zeus to grant him eternal youth as well. So Zeus fulfilled Eos' ill-expressed wish and Tithonos did get to live forever but forever becoming older and increasingly frail. Eventually, Tithonos had shrunk down into the form of an immortal cicada, begging for death to take him, taking up an unenviable place between 'men and gods: ageing like men, deathless like gods' (King, 1986, p. 17). Thus, the idea of immortality without eternal youth—of eternal ageing without death—is looked upon as an extremely negative prospect, inspiring the hope that there may be some secret way of rejuvenating people indefinitely, even if one must accept the inevitability of eventual death.

One central myth in this context is that of the 'Fountain of Youth', an important cultural gestalt in classical mythology, and a particularly strong theme in the work of Herodotus (fifth century BCE). The fountain returns youth to old people who drink from or bathe in it. The legend returned to prominence in the sixteenth century, when Juan Ponce de León, first Governor of Puerto Rico, allegedly began a search for the Fountain of Youth on behalf of the Spanish Crown. Although his quest was ultimately unsuccessful, he did manage to discover Florida in 1513. His search provided the title for an influential study published several centuries later, Carol Ryff's review on successful ageing: 'Beyond Ponce de León and Life Satisfaction: New Directions in Quest of Successful Ageing' (Ryff, 1989).

The Renaissance era also witnessed the emergence of more realistic ways of achieving a long and healthy life. Italian nobleman Alvise (Luigi) Cornaro argued in his book *The Sure and Certain Method of Attaining a Long and Healthful Life* (1550) that people could influence both the duration and quality of their lives as they grew older (Haber, 2004). The recipe for his realist Fountain of Youth was moderation in everything as a pathway to retaining one's vital energy up to very old age. Cornaro, by following his own advice, was to live to the age of 98. Interestingly, Cornaro saw age and ageing not as enemies to be combatted, but as an integral part of the course of human life course worthy of great reverence. Among the reasons he gave for appreciating old age were the wisdom and insight that it brought into life in general, as well as the opportunity to serve the community that these virtues provided. Cornaro argued that it was the responsibility of the individual to lead a good life up into very old age, just as many protagonists of successful ageing do today. *The Sure and Certain Method* continued to be republished right up until the nineteenth century, running to more than 50 editions. As a side note, doges—rulers of Venice between the seventh and eighteenth century— were almost all older men, not infrequently above the age of 80 years. As Finlay (1978) resumed in his in-depth analysis of the Venetian gerontocracy: 'Stability and harmony were virtues to be placed before the uncertain attractions of novelty and contention (. . .). Venice's governors enjoyed a justified reputation for being temperate, prudent, and unimaginative' (p. 178).

With the emergence of modern medicine in the nineteenth century, the positive notion of a good and meaningful later life began to be displaced by another that saw ageing as a disease to be resented and feared—and to be cured through the use of new medical treatments (Haber, 2004). Austrian physician Ignatz Nascher (1863–1944), the founder of geriatric medicine, remarked at the beginning of the twentieth century: 'It is impossible to draw a sharp line between health and disease in old age' (Nascher, 1910, p. 94). In this vein, several scientists, among them Austrian physiologist Eugen Steinach (1861–1944), Russian–French biologist Élie Metchnikoff (1845–1916), and American veterinary physiologist and pharmacologist Charles E. Stevens (1927–2008), argued for interventions in diet and hygiene in order to slow the process of ageing, or even eliminate it completely. At the risk of overstating the connection with the present, one might assert that the basic assumptions of these experiments—while their methods were very different—are not so far removed from the philosophy guiding more recent 'anti-ageing medicine' (Klatz & Goldman, 1997; see also Binstock, 2003).

In summary, the idea of living a long (or even eternal) life without accumulating age-related infirmities along the way can be set among that small set of cultural ideas that have retained their power across the millennia of human existence (Wahl, in press). However, it was only in the twentieth century that the quest for 'successful ageing' became a central, recurrent topic in scientific research.

Emergence of the concept 'successful ageing' in gerontology

After a number of early treatments, particularly those provided by Robert J. Havighurst (Havighurst, 1961, 1963; Havighurst & Albrecht, 1953), the final breakthrough within gerontology in the use of the term 'successful ageing' came with the publication in *Science* of an article by geriatrician Jack W. Rowe and psychologist and social scientist Robert L. Kahn (Rowe & Kahn, 1987). The same term was also used in the title of a much-cited anthology by researchers into ageing Paul Baltes and Margret Baltes (Baltes & Baltes, 1990b), whose aim was to further develop and demarcate Rowe and Kahn's conception, treating it mainly through the lens of the social and behavioural sciences.

In the wake of this early work, it is satisfying to see the large number of publications in more recent gerontology dedicated to publicizing and discussing the concept of successful ageing. Two important publications by Jack Rowe and Robert Kahn merit particular mention: an article in *The Gerontologist* (Rowe & Kahn, 1997), which up until June 2020 has been cited more than 1700 times (Web of Science), and a popular-science book, published probably not coincidentally in the Random House 'Large Print Series' to make it attractive to wider audiences, including to older adults themselves (Rowe & Kahn, 1998). It was through such publications that the term 'successful ageing' achieved a firm foothold in North American ageing research. However, these publications inspired disapproval and criticism (Katz & Calasanti, 2015). Full special issues of at least two flagship journals in gerontology—*The Gerontologist* (2015) and the *Journal of Gerontology* (2017)—explicitly addressed the concept of successful ageing and its ambitions and ambivalences. The criticisms provoked, in particular by Rowe and Kahn's model (Rowe & Kahn, 1997, 2015), addressed a broad range of issues from questioning the term 'successful' to missing components (e.g. well-being, spirituality) to accusations of blaming groups of older adults for not ageing successfully and nurturing elite thinking in gerontology.

In what direction are we heading with this book?

The notion of successful ageing has not only been one of the most successful, but also one of the most controversial concepts of ageing research over the last 60 years. Attempts to uncover the secret of successful ageing have often resembled something like a quest for the Golden Fleece. And that quest continues within contemporary gerontology—so far with no end in sight. And yet every treatment of the idea of successful ageing is faced with a challenge from the very term itself. On the one hand, the expression draws attention to the achievements of modern science, seeming to promise a disease-free later life and old age. Visions of how ageing in the future might further improve may be moved from unattainable longings to real scenarios. On the other hand, it might well be argued that using the term puts up a considerable barrier in itself; its very utterance can elicit immediate rejection, so hyperbolic do its implicit claims seem. Moreover, characterizing certain avenues into old age as 'successful' implies the existence of other 'unsuccessful' ones. Does it really make sense to think of frailty and dementia as a 'failure' of ageing, for example? Such questions illustrate how the ambition of the concept 'successful ageing' continues to be burdened with pronounced ambivalence.

This book argues that definitions of successful ageing largely depend on conflicting normative decisions. The neglect of the value systems behind these decisions has hindered any broad consensus as to what 'successful ageing' actually entails in practice. Moreover, strategies for promoting successful ageing may be expected to differ depending both on the definition one choses for the concept and on the relevant cultural–political–institutional context. Pursuing such aims as enhancing the physical capacity of older people or promoting their active engagement in society will likely rely on strategies quite different to measures aimed at fostering subjective well-being. In addition, a complex interaction exists between such differing policies on priorities in successful ageing and the wide variety of political and institutional systems in place in different countries. Actions aimed at modifying habits such as a sedentary lifestyle, for example, may conflict with one's subjective well-being and evoke resistance to leave decade-long established comfort zones, although they might promote physical and cognitive health. In any case, the contents of this book fully accepts Havighurst's insight that treating and implementing successful ageing always requires 'a value judgment on which people will be bound to disagree' (Havighurst, 1963, p. 299).

So, what *is* successful ageing? And how can it be achieved through individual initiative, focused efforts, and social policy? Or should we abandon the term up front and move on to other important discourses in ageing science? This monograph sets out to provide an overview of the various attempts that have been made to answer these questions. In view of the fact that Rowe and Kahn's model of successful ageing has already been subjected to thorough criticism (Katz & Calasanti, 2015), and that a wide variety of definitions of successful ageing have emerged over the years (Depp & Jeste, 2006), this book sets three goals for itself:

(1) to describe the various models used to define successful ageing and to provide not only a broader conceptual viewpoint to increase awareness of the complexity, richness, and ambition of the concept, but also of the ambivalences connected with it;

(2) to anchor the concept of successful ageing at the micro (individual), meso, and macro analytic levels of human development and ageing, and to present research capable of speaking to these three levels, an essential task in reaching an understanding of successful ageing and of the concepts used in its application;

(3) to discuss the usefulness of the concept in guiding policy and in informing the work of senior citizen organizations and other non-governmental institutions concerned with ageing societies across the globe.

Importantly, we aim to give an equally strong voice both to the ambitions of and ambivalences in the concept of successful ageing. However, we also strive to reconcile those ambitions and ambivalences, especially by counteracting any exclusion of any group of older adults without giving up the term successful ageing. If human frailty in later life is not given a fair chance of being considered within a range of notions of successful ageing, then the application of the concept 'successful ageing' may produce more harm than good in ageing science and practice. We argue that ageing research needs to consider a family of models of successful ageing anchored in a variety of value systems and philosophical traditions. Hence, we claim for 'controlled pluralism' as a key to further the discourse on successful ageing. Putting it differently, and touching again on Havighurst's (1963) claim that debates on successful ageing require 'a value judgment on which people will be bound to disagree', we argue that it would be unhelpful in conceptualizations of successful ageing to engage in something like a search for any Golden Fleece. Instead, it comes with much more heuristic value to be keenly aware of the differing values and norms that underlie the various models of successful ageing available to us—and then to come to a value judgement that agrees with one rather than another model, depending on a whole gamut of conditions. These may include the fundamental biological processes of ageing, individual resources, and goals in life, as well as spatial, socio-economic, political, and cultural contexts. We start by discussing our subject matter from the perspective of biogerontology.

2

Biological perspectives on successful ageing

Suresh I. S. Rattan

Biogerontologists most commonly describe ageing and old age as the process by which and the period during which a person experiences progressive decline, loss, and failure of their biological structures and functioning (Fulop et al., 2010; Rattan, 2015). This view of ageing is further reinforced by what are often referred to as the hallmarks of ageing at molecular, biochemical, and cellular levels, within which functional loss, impairment, and dysregulation are the prominent features (López-Otín et al., 2013). From a biological perspective, the lifetime of an organism can be represented as being divided into roughly two phases: a first phase of birth, growth, development, maturation, and reproduction; and the second phase of post-reproductive survival until the individual's eventual death. In evolutionary terms, the first period of life is referred to as a species' essential lifespan, the portion of life necessary and sufficient for the continuation of future generations (Rattan, 2000). The essential lifespan of a species has evolved through genetic selection and regulation via hundreds of genes involved in basic metabolic and maintenance functions, including DNA repair, protein repair and turnover, antioxidant defences, nutritional sensing, and so on. Such essential processes, also known as the unfolding of longevity-assurance genes (Jazwinski, 1998) or vitagenes (Rattan, 1998), determine a biological entity's overall ability to survive. This ability of a living system can be conceptualized via the notion of the 'homeodynamic space' available to it (Petrov, 2007; Rattan, 2014).

Three fundamental characteristics of an organism's homeodynamic space are its stress tolerance, damage control, and ability for constant remodelling and adaptation, all of which are essential to that individual's health and survival during its essential lifespan. However, during the period of survival beyond that point, progressive shrinkage of the homeodynamic space, owing to the accumulation of molecular damage, will result in physiological impairment, disease, and eventual death

(Demirovic & Rattan, 2013; Rattan, 1995, 2015). The text that follows provides a brief overview of the nature of the homeodynamic space, some of the reasons for its decline during the ageing process, and the possibilities available for its regulation and modulation in an effort to achieve successful ageing from a biological point of view.

Homeodynamic space

The concept of homeodynamics refines and expands upon the traditional term 'homeostasis', a notion based in the paradigm of the 'body as a machine' (Cannon, 1929, 1939). However, homeostasis does not sufficiently account for the dynamic nature of the information and interaction networks that underlie complex biological systems (Nicholson, 2019; Sholl & Rattan, 2019). The term homeodynamics therefore encompasses the fact that, unlike machines, the internal conditions of biological systems are not permanently fixed, are not at equilibrium, but are rather under constant dynamic regulation with constant interaction between their various levels of organization (Nicholson, 2019; Sholl & Rattan, 2019; Yates, 1994). The concept of homeodynamic space takes in the dynamic and interactive abilities of a biological system to survive and meet the demands of its constantly challenging internal and external milieu (Demirovic & Rattan, 2013; Petrov, 2007; Rattan, 2014).

The main biomarkers of the homeodynamic space are: (1) stress responses, that is, how far a system can tolerate and manage perturbations induced by intrinsic and extrinsic stressors; (2) damage control systems—the repair processes that switch on after cell damage; and (3) constant remodelling—the overall ability to tolerate, compensate, and adapt at both cellular and physiological level (Demirovic & Rattan, 2013; Rattan, 2020a; Sholl & Rattan, 2019). Table 2.1 provides examples of the biological processes that comprise these characteristics within the homeodynamic space.

The homeodynamic space describes one's overall ability, which can be analysed as a set of phenotypic parameters (robustness and resilience, for example) of an individual's or subsystem's performance in the face of a specific perturbation (Rattan, 2020a; Sholl & Rattan, 2019). This ability and its biomarkers correspond to the measurable changes that help distinguish the relevant parameters from one another and evaluate their individual contributions to the homeodynamic space (Rattan, 2020a; Sholl & Rattan, 2019). Thus, the notion of homeodynamic space is not merely a theoretical concept,

Table 2.1. Mechanistic and measurable biomarkers in the homeodynamic space

Homeodynamic characteristic	Examples of the processes involved
Stress response	DNA repair response, anti-oxidative response, nutritional stress response, autophagy, inflammatory response
Damage control	Macromolecular turnover and repair, free radical scavenging, detoxification
Constant remodelling	Cellular turnover and programmed cell death (apoptosis), immune system remodelling, bone remodelling, tissue regeneration, thermoregulation

but may be taken as a measure of an individual's biological health and/or success (Rattan, 2020a).

The survival of a newly born organism will depend absolutely on its possessing a certain range of homeodynamic space. Although its size may not yet be fully quantified or quantifiable, there are several factors that shape it; factors that begin to make themselves felt as early as in embryonic and fetal life (Rattan, 2020a). A lack of optimal nutrition, for example, or the presence of infectious agents such as toxic chemicals/drugs, and high levels of stress hormones in the blood of the mother negatively affect the growth and adaptive capacities of the developing embryo; and such influences may have lifelong negative effects on the health and survival of a newborn (Vaiserman, 2019). Similarly, malnutrition, social distress, and infectious disease in early childhood and adolescence leave a mark that can last throughout a person's adult lifespan, usually manifested as an increased incidence of metabolic disease, including obesity, diabetes, cardiovascular failure, neurodegenerative diseases, and general frailty (Vaiserman, 2019).

Normal processes of growth, development, and maturation further extend and strengthen the homeodynamic space available to organisms, enabling them biologically to survive and reproduce as ordained by the evolutionary history of their species. For example, species that mature fast, begin reproducing early and have large numbers of progeny at each round of reproduction will generally have a short essential lifespan and a more restricted homeodynamic space. Among mammals, rats, mice, hamsters, and gerbils provide examples of such species. In contrast, species with slow maturation, late onset of reproduction, and small numbers of progeny generally coincides with a long essential lifespan and a large homeodynamic space (Finch, 2009; Finch & Kirkwood, 2000). Our species, together with a few others, such as elephants and whales, are examples of animals with long essential lifespan and a larger homeodynamic space.

It is essential to point out here that a biological understanding of life and its evolution would assert that evolution neither aims for nor requires that systems be perfect (Finch & Kirkwood, 2000; Holliday, 2007; Rattan, 2006). Infidelity in copying and imperfections in biochemical processes produce deviations from and dysregulations within biological systems, providing the very stage upon which evolution occurs (Finch & Kirkwood, 2000; Holliday, 2007). The three components of the homeodynamic space (stress response processes, damage control mechanisms, and constant remodelling) are not perfect: they are prone to the occurrence and accumulation of molecular damage, leading to functional decline (Holliday, 2007; Rattan, 2006). Such imperfections in molecular processes, together with the progressive increase in entropy ordained by the second law of thermodynamics, provide the ultimate cause of the failure, collapse, and demise of all living systems (Demetrius & Legendre, 2013; Hayflick, 2007). The maximum lifespan of an individual and the timing of that individual's death are only indirectly determined by the limitations of the genes ensuring longevity that provide the homeodynamic space and not at all by any self-destructing and ageing-triggering gerontogenes that may be present (Demirovic & Rattan, 2013; Rattan, 1995, 2015).

Shrinkage of homeodynamic space
as we age

During an individual's essential lifespan, the occurrence and accumulation of some level of molecular damage at the cellular level has little or no obvious harmful consequences for the physiological functioning and survival of an organism. This is because the scale of day-to-day damage generally falls within the capacity of the homeodynamic space to tolerate, repair, or remove the damaged DNA, RNA, protein, and other molecules. However, during the period beyond an organism's essential lifespan, the accumulation of molecular damage becomes far more significant, eventually overwhelming the ability of the organism's imperfect homeodynamic space to counteract it (Rattan, 2008). Some examples of molecular damage thought to increase during the ageing process are listed below.

- Mutations, which may occur spontaneously due to errors in DNA replication, or be induced by external agents such as ultraviolet radiation and mutagenic toxins, are irreversible alterations in the DNA sequencing of an individual's genome.
- Epimutations—the spontaneous or induced reversible changes in the nucleotide bases of the DNA making up an individual's genome and their chromosomal histone proteins, by the addition or removal of particular chemical entities (methyl and acetyl groups, respectively), alter the extent of gene expression.
- Loss of telomere DNA at the end of chromosomes during DNA duplication, destabilizing the genome and disrupting cell division.
- Oxidative and sugar-induced modification of amino acids in proteins, leading to protein misfolding and aggregations of insoluble proteins both inside and outside the cells.

Accumulated molecular damage causes a shrinkage in the homeodynamic space, and manifests itself as a progressive decline in the affected individual's physiological capacities, in increasing functional impairments and frailty, and in the emergence of a range of chronic pathologies. Ideally, from a biological perspective, successful ageing would therefore entail the prevention, treatment, and/or elimination of all the above features of the ageing process. Maintaining, recovering, and strengthening the homeodynamic space throughout one's life, and especially in old age, would seem to be a necessary condition for a biologically successful healthy ageing process.

Homeodynamics and health

Health is often described either as the absence of one or more diseases, or as a rather undefined notion of well-being. However, defining health via the concept of homeodynamic space can make a connection between the functionality of a biological system and its successful survival (Rattan, 2020a). In this context, a measure widely accepted and employed in practice in the medical, social–behavioural, and health sciences is the concept of 'activities of daily living' (ADL; Wiener et al., 1990). Combining ADL with a set of other physiological and biochemical measurements is a useful approach in the task of defining, measuring, and quantifying the relative state of health of an individual (Gao et al., 2016; Spector & Fleishman, 1998).

Health could therefore be defined as a state of absolute physical and mental independence in one's ADL (Demirovic & Rattan, 2013), although such an idealized state is clearly impossible to achieve fully. Thus, in effect, being healthy means having a sufficient level of physical and mental independence in one's ADL—a state that may vary widely but is nevertheless open to being established objectively (Demirovic & Rattan, 2013; Rattan, 2020a; Sholl & Rattan, 2019). Furthermore, such a pragmatic definition of health will tend to allow and/or encourage the use of all kinds of medical, nutritional, technological and other external strategies (including social and mental interventional approaches) in the effort to maintain, facilitate, recover, and enhance people's functional health. Biologically successful ageing will thus entail having sufficient independence in one's ADL. Sufficient independence in ADL can even be achieved while living with chronic diseases with the help of biomedical, psychological, technological, and societal interventions.

Implications for interventions towards successful ageing

The approach one takes towards interventions to achieve successful ageing is influenced by one's understanding of ageing either as a disease in need of treatment or as a condition emerging from basic life processes, which, in turn, are, to some extent, subject to modulation. If we consider ageing as an emergent phenotype caused by imperfections in the homeodynamic space rather than by the predetermined programme of a variety of life-limiting and death-causing mechanisms, such a view will modify the interventional approach from one involving 'anti-ageing' strategies to one in which the aim will be to achieve 'healthy' or 'successful ageing'.

This change of approach will also have major consequences for interventions relating to successful ageing. Among the most prevalent biomedical approaches to anti-ageing is a set of interventions often referred to as piecemeal remedies. The basic logic behind them involves limiting oneself to 'fixing what's broke'; its interventions range from tissue and/or organ repair or transplantation to targeted treatments using stem cells, rejuvenation by transfusing young blood or plasma and the elimination of senescent cells using potential senolytic compounds (Rattan, 2020a). Although such interventions will often be life-saving in acute situations, their benefits are often transient and limited, frequently requiring repeated application.

In contrast to the limited results of single target-based interventions, the approaches that have successfully shown significant health-promoting effects tend to be far more holistic. Physical exercise, dietary habits, sleep, and maintaining social and mental engagement seem to form the pillars of good health and longer life. Interventions of this type tend to have multiple and cumulative effects. Although changes in specific biological markers can be shown from each of such holistic interventions, the effectiveness of any of them cannot be reduced to any single or even limited number of targets. For example, the whole-body health benefits of regular moderate exercise (Biernat & Piatkowska, 2018) and of restricted food intake (Fontana & Partridge, 2015) cannot be replicated by any targeted stimulation of any one or limited number of molecular markers or processes associated with them. The same applies to individual components of foodstuffs and other natural or synthetic compounds that may be shown to have one or multiple targets of action at the molecular level. Most often they either fail to provide results beneficial to one's physiological well-being and health in real life or are accompanied by substantial detrimental side effects on one's health (Vaiserman et al., 2016).

One promising holistic interventionary approach towards achieving successful ageing worth mentioning is the use of the phenomenon of hormesis—the beneficial, life-supporting effects that result from the cellular and organismic responses to repeated or transient exposure to mild stresses (Rattan, 2020b). Moderate physical exercise provides the main paradigm of stress-induced physiological hormesis. One important observation that has emerged from studies of physiological hormesis is that a single stressor, such as heat, exercise, or fasting can strengthen overall homeodynamics and enhance other abilities, including cognition, hormonal balance, immune response, memory, resilience, and robustness (Rattan, 2020b). Strengthening and maintaining the homeodynamic space is an achievable goal for successful ageing, from a biological point of view at least.

3
A taxonomy of successful ageing conceptions

Before studying the topic of successful ageing in depth, one first needs to define what is meant by the term—and in doing so to make a *normative decision* on what the desirable endpoints of ageing should be. Hence, at this point, we enter the sphere of value judgements on what successful ageing should look like. Should we strive to achieve immaculate developmental outcomes over one's lifespan, directing our efforts to minimizing the damaging effects of growing old, and calling the result 'successful ageing'? Or should we embrace the diversity of ageing? Developmental trajectories in the second half of one's lifetime are likely to look quite different from individual to individual. Some might enjoy bodily and mental fitness until the very end, while others become frail and dependent towards the end of their lives. Is it possible that 'successful ageing' lies beyond bodily functioning, consisting rather of the accumulation of wisdom and serenity? Or, supposing we accept frailty as part of ageing, might we consider the provision of adequate care with the aim of supporting the dignity of each person until the end of their lives as 'successful ageing'?

Questions like these touch on some very basic ideas and values of what it means to lead a good life. We should therefore take a look at the various philosophical traditions that describe such a good life (Hakim, 2016). Doing so makes it clear that what constitutes a good life will depend on one's philosophical orientation. In this chapter, we suggest organizing existing models of successful ageing according to five philosophical perspectives[1] on what a good life constitutes:

- pragmatic approach;
- hedonic approach;

---

[1] Despite none of us being a philosopher, we feel that there is need to rely on philosophical approaches to analyse the normative foundations of different views on successful ageing. Although we see our limitations, we hope to do justice to a philosophical approach on successful ageing.

- eudaimonic approach;
- capability-related approach;
- care ethics-based approach.

Based on these philosophical definitions of a good life, we examine the implications of each perspective in reaching an understanding of successful ageing. We are not saying that these models of successful ageing offer a fully comprehensive approach to capture the concept. However, we do argue that the five perspectives provide a heuristically fruitful route towards classifying and comparing existing approaches in the current literature on successful ageing and that it also has appeal in practice and policy.

Pragmatic model of successful ageing

Pragmatism is a philosophical tradition that emphasizes practical use and success as a guideline for the evaluation of concepts, ideas, theories, and life (Dewey, 1931; Rescher, 1999). It is not the search for truth that occupies pragmatism, but the task of changing the world for the good of humankind. It sees ideas as tools for altering reality. Hence, pragmatism does not pose the question what life is, but rather tries to answer questions about what can be done to make life worth living. What this means for individuals is that the important thing is to empower individual agency (i.e. the ability to make choices and the capacity to act accordingly). In other words, a good life consists of leading an active life, and altering one's circumstances in order to better fit one's goals and plans. It is of note that John Dewey contributed an introductory chapter to the first highly interdisciplinary oriented handbook on the topic of the science of ageing, Cowdry's *Problems of Ageing* (Cowdry, 1939). Toward the end of his introductory comments, Dewey unfolds his pragmatic view of the possibilities open to human ageing by telling the reader: 'When we shall envisage social relations and institutions in the light of the contribution they are capable of making to continued growth, when we are capable of criticizing those which exist on the ground of the ways in which they arrest and deflect processes of growth, we shall be on our way to a solution of the moral and psychological problems of human ageing' (Cowdry, 1939, p. xxxiii).

Moving to modern ageing science, one of the most prominent models of successful ageing, the model of geriatrician John Rowe and social scientist Robert Kahn, is deeply rooted in the tradition of pragmatism (Rowe

& Kahn, 1987, 1997). In brief, successful ageing in the pragmatic tradition consists of preserving individual agency into old age, based on promoting and protecting one's health, functioning, and participation in society. The starting point of Rowe and Kahn's model of successful ageing is the large variability—a variability that increases with advancing age—among older adults, a phenomenon that implies that some people do age more favourably than others. To illustrate the importance of this insight, Rowe and Kahn use tangible labels for the various ranges within this distribution. The term 'successful ageing' is applied to ageing trajectories up at the top of the distribution in terms of health, functional capacity, and activity, while trajectories at the bottom, characterized by illness and functional impediments, fall under the label 'pathological ageing'. Trajectories towards the mid-range of the distribution are labelled 'usual ageing'. As Rowe and Kahn also state, there is a 'need for interdisciplinary studies of the factors that determine the trajectory of function with advancing age . . . explaining the heterogeneity of older people with respect to those functions' (Rowe & Kahn, 1987, p. 148).

Rowe and Kahn define 'successful ageing as including three main components: low probability of disease and disease-related disability, high cognitive and physical functional capacity, and active engagement with life' (1997, p. 433). Two of these components—a low probability of illness and a high level of (cognitive and physical) functioning—provide the prerequisites that permit a third component: active engagement with life. Staying healthy, keeping fit, and remaining active in society and striving to change the world all the way into old age is deemed to constitute successful ageing, while ageing in ill health and without the capacity to participate actively in society is not.

Individual strategies for successful ageing, as defined by Rowe and Kahn include, for instance, pursuing a healthy lifestyle (Fries et al., 2011) and activating one's own latent reserve capacities (Baltes et al., 2006). More recently, Rowe and Kahn (2015) called for research into what they named 'Successful Ageing 2.0'. As societies continue to grow older, ageing research needs to analyse policies that allow societies to deal successfully with the benefits and risks of demographic change (i.e. policies that foster productivity, cohesion, resilience, and sustainability in ageing societies). Rowe and Kahn make the claim that 'successful ageing at the societal level will obviously facilitate successful ageing at the level of the individual, and, most likely, vice versa' (2015, p. 2).

Rowe and Kahn's model provides the background for most ongoing discussions on successful ageing, but it has attracted quite a few criticisms. Firstly, it has been pointed out that the model is exclusive. Hank and colleagues, using data from the Survey of Health, Ageing and Retirement in Europe (SHARE) study—the best survey study currently available to represent ageing across Europe—found large differences between European countries in the proportion of older people ageing successfully according to the criteria of Rowe and Kahn's conception (Hank, 2011). Comparing age groups, McLaughlin and colleagues used the Health and Retirement Study (HRS), one of the world's most robust survey data sets, and observed dwindling rates of successful ageing in older age groups (McLaughlin et al., 2010). These findings make it apparent that not all people will age successfully, illustrating the dark side of successful ageing: individuals whose conditions do not fulfil the criteria of health, functioning, and activity must necessarily be counted as failures. And as this flip side of successful ageing is not considered at all in the model, large sections of the ageing population remain simply out of sight. This partial blindness is not a random effect: it depends heavily on social class. To a considerable extent, education, income, and wealth determine the probability of a person ageing successfully. In other words: individuals from lower social strata are less likely to age successfully than their more fortunate peers from the upper echelons of society (Hank, 2011). Premature mortality is also strongly related to socio-economic status (SES). A British study found that more than one-third of all premature deaths were attributable to inequality in SES, with tuberculosis, opioid use, HIV, psychoactive drugs use, viral hepatitis, and obesity playing a dominant role in causes of premature death (Lewer et al., 2020).

Secondly, the model places the greatest burden of responsibility for reaching successful ageing on individuals themselves, neglecting the role of societal structures and inequalities. It has been argued that any theorizing on successful ageing should acknowledge 'the interplay between lives and the complementary dynamic of structural change' (Riley, 1998, p. 151). Social structures may not only act as facilitators, but also as impediments to successful ageing.

A third criticism points to the fact that Rowe and Kahn's model does not consider the subjective views of older people themselves. The model thus runs the risk of imposing a definition of good life in old age that is not necessarily shared by older people themselves. Several studies have shown that older people tend to define successful ageing more broadly and on a more multidimensional basis than Rowe and Kahn's model, with the former including well-being and positive affect in their assessments (Jopp et al., 2015).

The multiple critiques of the model is to some extent a consequence of its fame. Rowe and Kahn's model is arguably the most influential of all models for successful ageing. It has been cited in a vast number of theoretical and empirical papers—and the impact of the term is still growing (Rowe & Carr, 2018, p. 1). As a *pars pro toto* for the vast literature, one might point to the aforementioned special issues of *The Gerontologist* (2015) and the *Journal of Gerontology* (2017). In any case, Rowe and Kahn's model provides the benchmark for other models of successful ageing to follow.

Hedonic model of successful ageing

In the tradition of hedonic philosophy, the notions of life satisfaction and happiness are seen as the yardsticks by which a good life should be measured (Lampe, 2015). Pursuing positive experiences (pleasure, happiness, and satisfaction) and avoiding negative experiences (depression, anger, and dissatisfaction) represent the core of that model. In contrast to pragmatist models, its focus is on one's subjective experience of the world rather than on any objective evaluation of one's capacities, activities, or contextual living conditions. The good life is in the eye of the beholder, and reasons to be happy and satisfied are as diverse as humankind itself.

According to this philosophical perspective (and in contrast to the pragmatic model), one cannot prescribe the meaning of successful ageing normatively: it is a judgement that lies exclusively in the hands of older individuals themselves. Havighurst's model of successful ageing is an early instance of the use of a hedonic approach to the concept (Havighurst, 1961, 1963). Of note, a ground-breaking article on how one might measure life satisfaction was published in the same year as Havighurst first suggested his model (Neugarten et al., 1961) in the first issue of *The Gerontologist*, the Gerontological Society of America's flagship journal for applied gerontology. His basic tenet appeals to the ineludibly normative character of discussions on successful ageing: 'a theory of successful ageing is an affirmation of certain values. Persons with different values of life in the later years will have different definitions and theories of successful ageing' (Havighurst, 1961, p. 12). The reasoning behind Havighurst's first attempt to unpack the complexity of life satisfaction was based on a multidimensional notion of the construct. Although one might well argue over the dimensions chosen by Havighurst at the time (i.e. zest vs apathy, resolution and fortitude, goodness of fit between desired and achieved goals, a positive self-image, and mood tone), it becomes clear that his view of life satisfaction is not dependent on any particular activity or environmental constellation. The 'zest vs apathy' dimension, for instance, relates to the enthusiasm a person feels towards their own activities, ideas, or social partners—and not to the particular activities that a person pursues, the particular ideas that a person holds or the size of their social network. A 'person who "just loves to sit home and knit" rates as high as the person who "loves to get out and meet people"' (Havighurst, 1961, p. 10). With respect to life goals, it is not the type or social acceptability of a goal that counts, but the goodness of fit between one's original plan and the final outcome. In Havighurst's words: 'High ratings [in respect to goodness of fit between desired and achieved goals] would go, for instance, to the man who says, "I've managed to keep out of jail" just as to the man who says, "I've managed to send all my kids through college"' (Havighurst, 1961, p. 11).

Hence, the hedonic approach tries to avoid making any a priori normative decisions on what counts as a good life—this can only be decided by ageing individuals themselves based on the extent of life satisfaction and happiness that it is possible for them to achieve. Accordingly, individuals who report a positive balance in their happiness/life satisfaction versus unhappiness/life dissatisfaction equation are classified as successful agers, while those for whom the balance is negative are not.

Over the decades, Havighurst's initial multidimensional approach to assessing successful ageing has often been reduced to the measurement of cognitive and affective well-being as proxies for successful ageing outcomes. An example of this simplified approach can be seen in definitions of subjective well-being made up of measurements of satisfaction (involving both global and domain-specific judgements on one's life) and affect (frequency of positive and negative emotions; see Diener, 2000). At its most extreme simplification, the hedonic approach has even been narrowed down in its operationalization to a single question, typically phrased as something like 'How satisfied are you with your life, all things considered?', a question contained, for example, in the German Socio-Economic Panel (SOEP; Gerstorf et al., 2008) and in other large-scale survey studies such as the World Value Survey (Oishi et al., 2009).

The hedonic approach acknowledges the great diversity among human beings and highlights their astonishing capacity to adapt to a wide range of living situations and critical life events. As advancing age is accompanied by losses—some of them irretrievable—this adaptive potential is a highly important aspect of the hedonic model. Humans tend to adjust to poor living situations and disruptive events by getting used to the new situation or by changing their reference standards—thus maintaining their life satisfaction (Brickman et al., 1978; Luhmann & Intelisano, 2018). It could well be that this ability is one mechanism behind what has been called the 'life satisfaction paradox of old age' (Staudinger et al., 1995): the observation that levels of satisfaction with life remain rather high as people grow older. This insight chimes well with the general hedonic approach: it is not one's objective situation which constitutes a good life, but one's subjective evaluation of it.

A problem with the hedonic approach relates to limitations on one's ability to adapt to differing circumstances. The hedonic approach attempts to disentangle one's objective living situation from one's subjective evaluation of that situation by arguing that such evaluations are not determined by the features of that situation, but rather by one's values. But this may be simply untrue of certain types of life event and in situations of destitution. Certain events, such as widowhood or repeated spells of unemployment, may have lasting effects on the life satisfaction of individuals, demonstrating the limits of the *hedonic treadmill* (Diener et al., 2006). According to the hedonic treadmill analogy, individuals are affected only temporarily by critical life events, eventually returning to their usual level of adaptation. In addition, there are some universal basic needs that simply must be met for everyone. If one's basic needs—for food and water, shelter, and clothing— remain unfulfilled, it seems inconceivable that any person could experience happiness and life satisfaction. With old age, chronic pain—an experience associated with low levels of life satisfaction—becomes an increasingly relevant factor. Hence, one of the basic tenets of the hedonic approach—that happiness can be found in the eye of the beholder—may not apply in extreme situations and in cases of severe loss.

Nevertheless, the hedonic approach has had in the past, and to a large extent still has, an enormous influence on ageing research, on practical interventions, and policy. Many empirical ageing studies, although they frequently do not appeal explicitly to a hedonic definition of successful ageing, often use subjective well-being as a central indicator of whether one is ageing well (e.g. George, 2010). Social indicators, such as the general satisfaction and happiness of an older population, also bear witness to the relevance of the hedonic approach for policy decisions. Last, but not least, a great many of us strive to continue to be happy and satisfied until late in life. However, empirical research has shown that life satisfaction fluctuates over one's life course, increasing from our middle years to early old age but declining from the age of about 70 onwards (Baird et al., 2010). Moreover, at the end of life a *terminal decline* of life satisfaction has empirically been found in that variability in life satisfaction can be better explained by distance from impending death compared to distance to birth (i.e. chronological age). Although pronounced heterogeneity exists in individual trajectories, life satisfaction continues to mark hedonic successful ageing until the very end of life (Gerstorf et al., 2010a).

Eudaimonic model of successful ageing

The goal of achieving wisdom and tranquillity of the mind is an ideal for a good life in the tradition of eudaimonic philosophy (Ryff, 1995, 2018). The concept of 'eudaimonia', a notion originating in Greek philosophy, means more than simply happiness or well-being: rather it should be interpreted as flourishing, development or self-actualization, hence as a notion that helps us to identify the sort of persons we should strive to be and the way we should strive to live (Hursthouse & Pettigrove, 2018). From this perspective, a good life does not depend on material success, health or happiness, but on internal virtues and moral integrity. Personal virtues are the essential character traits of an individual, including things like honesty, mercy, or dependability. These virtues form an integral part of what it is to live a desirable, worthwhile life.

The last phase of life brings new developmental challenges, and coping with them requires reaching new levels of personal growth. This notion of a good life in old age is quite different from the wish to remain healthy, fit, and active for as long as possible (following the pragmatic model) or to remain happy and satisfied until the end of life (pursuing the hedonic model). Adopting a developmental perspective on eudaimonic well-being means searching 'for the higher, more differentiated growth processes that occur with ageing rather than examining essentially nondevelopmental dimensions (e.g., life satisfaction)' (Ryff, 1982, p. 210). Insights into existential questions of life and death, reflecting on one's own biography with its successes and failures, loyalties and betrayals, loves and hates as belonging to one's own life, and giving advice to the generations to come—such achievements are the ideals of the eudaimonic approach to successful ageing, an approach that even acknowledges the potential of negative experiences to exert a positive developmental influence on those who suffer them.

Life-course scholar and psychodynamic clinician Erik H. Erikson's model of 'psychosocial stages' is the most prominent example of a successful ageing model in the eudaimonic tradition (Erikson, 1963, 1968). Over the course of their lives, individuals are confronted with ever-new developmental tasks as they arise along the way. From the beginning to the end, a person experiences a sequential series of challenges arising through the tension between their developing individual needs and the prevailing societal expectations. These developmental tasks generate psychosocial crises that the individual needs to resolve and that will result in a positive or negative outcome for one's subsequent personality development, depending on how successfully one copes with them. The very first developmental tasks arise all the way back in infancy and childhood ('trust vs mistrust', 'autonomy vs shame', 'initiative vs guilt', 'industry vs inferiority'). Adolescence is characterized by the most famous developmental task identified in Eriksonian theory: 'Identity formation' (vs 'identity confusion'). The periods of young and middle adulthood are marked by the crises of 'intimacy vs isolation' and 'generativity vs stagnation'.

The developmental challenge posed by old age is, according to Erikson's view, the acceptance of one's lifetime at a point in time at which past life has been lived, major decisions made in younger years cannot be reversed, and remaining lifetime does not allow for a new life. By Erikson's account, the psychosocial crisis in old age is delineated by the endpoints 'ego integrity vs despair'. Expressed in Erikson's (1963) own words this last developmental task concerns 'the acceptance of one's one and only life cycle as something that had to be and that, by necessity, permitted of no substitutions' (p. 268). Successful ageing consists of accepting one's biography, with all its successes and failures, as one's own unique life. Later, Joan and Erik Erikson wrote about the developmental challenges of very old age: 'Old age in one's eighties and nineties brings with it new demands, reevaluations, and daily difficulties' (Erikson & Erikson, 1997, p. 105). During this ninth stage, all the psychosocial crises of the eight previous stages need to be dealt with once more, but with the relationship between the two poles reversed. For instance, while the infant develops basic trust, the very old person develops a mistrust of his or her own capabilities. Older individuals who have the capacity to accept these facts, to develop a level of ego integrity and to acquire a certain wisdom and insight into life, are seen as examples of successful agers, while older people lost in sorrow or despair are not.

Another example of an eudaimonic approach to successful ageing is Carol Ryff's theory of personal growth (Ryff, 1989). This approach integrates lifespan developmental theories, clinical theories of personal growth, and mental health perspectives. According to this perspective, successful ageing consists of advanced progression along six developmental dimensions: self-acceptance; positive relations with others; autonomy; environmental mastery; purpose in life; and personal growth. Contrasting 'high and low scorers' over these dimensions, Ryff describes what successful ageing consists of from this perspective. On the personal growth dimension, for instance, successful ageing means that the person 'has a feeling of continued development and sees self as growing and expanding', while unsuccessful ageing means that a person 'has a sense of personal stagnation and lacks a sense of improvement or expansion over time' (Ryff, 1989, p. 46). At the empirical level, Ryff and Keyes (1995) found that the personal growth and purpose in life dimensions were at their lowest in older adults as compared to individuals in young adulthood or midlife. In contrast, positive relations, environmental mastery, self-acceptance, and autonomy were either at their peak in old age or remained relatively stable over one's lifetime. Apparently, there is pronounced multidirectionality in successful ageing indicators according to the eudaimonic perspective, and not all indicators of a eudaimonic understanding of successful ageing may necessarily point to an increase or steady maintenance of such indicators over one's lifetime. In other words, age-related loss is not necessarily inimical to successful ageing.

The intellectual appeal of the eudaimonic approach is based on the fact that it goes beyond such single dimensions as health or life satisfaction. It also shows the complex and rich challenges and multifaceted nature of old age as a phase of life, and illustrates how successful ageing is not always easy for the ageing individual to construct actively. What the approach does reveal, however, is the most radically normative foundation, as compared to both the preceding approaches and the ones to follow. It relies on theoreticians setting the criteria for successful personal growth by making a judgement on what the good life in old age *should* look like. Although this problem has been acknowledged in the eudaimonic tradition (e.g. Ryff, 1989, p. 49), this normative orientation in eudaimonic models for successful ageing may be seen as too restrictive when it comes to development in old age.

Another problem with this approach is the fact that one needs cognitive abilities to recognize and solve developmental tasks, to excel in creating purpose in one's life, and to strive for personal fulfilment and growth (Baltes et al., 2006). As cognitive decline can frequently be observed in very old age and dementia-related disorders are far from uncommon, the consequence of this is that successful ageing is inaccessible for a considerable number of people suffering problems with their capacity to remember, reason, or reflect. Nevertheless, eudaimonic models provide a fascinating variant of defining what a good life in old age consists of: providing the grounds upon which other conceptions in this realm, such as gerotranscendence theory, have been formulated (e.g. Tornstam, 2005; see also Diehl & Wahl, 2020).

Capability-related model of successful ageing

In the capability-related approach to successful ageing, the question of key importance is the following: Who is responsible for a good life? In the philosophical traditions discussed up until now, it is the individual who is accountable for staying fit (in the pragmatic model), striving for happiness (the hedonic model), or aspiring to wisdom (the eudaimonic model). But individuals do not live in isolation. They live with family and friends, in villages or cities, in specific geographical territories, and under specific climatic conditions. Moreover, individuals form part of societies with particular modes of production, social inequalities, and social policies. All these contextual conditions facilitate (or impede) to a very great extent their prospects for a good life.

Starting from these considerations, Amartya Sen's capability-based approach to a good life emphasizes precisely such structures of opportunity and impediment (Sen, 1993). As Sen states, the capability approach concerns itself with the opportunities for an individual to 'achieve various valuable functionings as a part of living' (1993, p. 30). His approach is based on three central concepts taken from the field of welfare economics: 'functionings', 'commodities', and 'capabilities'. It is important to note that the meanings of these terms differ considerably from those used in the standard terminology of the social and behavioural sciences. As Sen uses the terms, 'functionings' may be equated with goals, 'commodities' with resources, and 'capabilities' with opportunity structures. Imagine, for instance, a person who likes to perform outdoor exercise (has a goal/functioning) and owns a bicycle (possesses a resource/commodity) but lives in an environment where no adequate cycle paths—necessary requirements for cycling—are available (i.e. the relevant opportunity/capability is absent). However, even if it is not possible for that person to reach her goal (exercising outdoors) through cycling, there may be other opportunity structures available to achieve the same goal, such as opportunities for jogging or walking. Thus, the combination of individual resources and environmental opportunity structures establishes a space of options for an individual to be or to do whatever she/he happens to value. The capability model's acknowledgement that individual values and ways to achieve them can differ tremendously fits very well with the pronounced heterogeneity as a key characteristic of old age: ageing individuals choose a huge diversity of sets of values in their pursuit of a good life. Hence, there must be multiple pathways towards a good life in old age.

These considerations have enormous consequences for the conceptualization of successful ageing. As we have already seen, the three models of successful ageing discussed so far (i.e. the pragmatic, the hedonic, and the eudaimonic models) have looked upon the concept as an individual achievement, neglecting the vastly varied opportunity structures that may restrict or broaden the avenues toward successful ageing. Looked at from the perspective of the capability approach, successful ageing is less of an achievement of the ageing individual alone than it is the result of an interaction between the individual and the opportunities and constraints within which that individual lives.

External factors, such as social networks, financial resources, or environmental supports are, in principle, relevant to all approaches to successful ageing. Still, the conceptualization of these factors differs between more individualistic as opposed to more inter-actionistic approaches. In individualistic approaches, external factors are seen as influencing the 'successful ageing outcome'. For instance, functional capacity, happiness, or personal growth (individualistically defined outcomes of successful ageing) may be influenced by social networks and social support (external factors). In contrast, the capability perspective is inter-actionalistic and conceptualizes external factors as *constitutive and co-constructing elements* of successful ageing, for instance by institutional structures, legal regulations, and policies. This accords well with a variety of gerontological traditions that start from the idea that a good life in old age is not an individual achievement alone. Prominent examples include the theory of social convoys (Antonucci et al., 2010; Kahn & Antonucci, 1980), environmental gerontology (Wahl & Gerstorf, 2018; Wahl & Weisman, 2003), or the theory of cumulate (dis)advantage (Dannefer, 2003; Ferraro & Shippee, 2009). These approaches to ageing research differ in many details, but they converge in one important point: they conceive the individual as being embedded—into social networks, physical environments, or social structures. This embeddedness into social, environmental, and societal contexts can be seen as opportunity structures (or impediments) for successful ageing.

Care-related model of successful ageing

In gerontology and geriatrics, discourse and research on frailty and dependency, on the one hand, and healthy and successful ageing, on the other, are very different strands of research, with only very few scientists working in both areas simultaneously. If, for instance, the connections between the terms 'successful ageing' and 'frailty' are discussed, the conversation among both worlds of ageing science is mostly carried on in terms of some underlying construct (e.g. functioning and fitness) involving two opposing poles— with successful ageing on one end and frailty on the other (e.g. Lowry et al., 2012; Rolfson, 2018). This is highly unsatisfactory, for two reasons.

The first argument refers to the sheer number of people who experience bodily and cognitive decline to such an extent that they require outside support and care. If the probability is high that a person is likely to experience a need of care over her lifetime, it does not seem reasonable to attribute this state as being the responsibility of an older person alone. Secondly, the loss of abilities and functions seems to be an integral part of the process of ageing. When one accepts the conviction that—despite all efforts in preventive healthcare—advanced age will be accompanied by irretrievable losses, it may be necessary to think about models of successful ageing that reach beyond simple worship of middle adulthood.

The interdependency between individuals, taken as one of the basic characteristics of being human, has been addressed in the feminist philosophical tradition of care ethics (Geissler & Pfau-Effinger, 2005; Tronto, 2014). In contrast to deontological ethics (in which decisions are based on rules) or consequentialism (where decisions are based on the results of actions), care ethics emphasizes the centrality of human relationship and cooperation to care for others. From this perspective the world is seen as 'comprised of relationships rather than of people standing alone, a world that coheres through human connection rather than through systems of rules' (Gilligan, 1982, p. 4). Hence, interdependency between people, dependency on one another, is not a deficiency that arises in old age, but a basic human characteristic whose expression—but not its fundamental nature—changes as one passes through the various phases of one's life.

Seen from the standpoint of care ethics, successful ageing is not the achievement of an autonomous ageing person resulting in good health, a broad spectrum of activity, and lots of social ties, but a process in which caregivers provide care in an attentive, responsible, and competent manner, and care receivers respond to these acts of support. Depending on the theoretical position a person holds, successful ageing might be defined as the fulfilment of individual needs, as the achievement of outcomes aspired to, or as the experience of appreciative and respectful interaction. Importantly, through the lens of care ethics successful ageing is again seen, similar to the capability model, as an important form of *co-construction* of an older person receiving care and another person who provides advice, help, support, and care. The joint endeavours of care receiver and caregiver are important, in their striving to maintain the self-determination and quality of life of an older person in need of care, even where such endeavours involve the use of long-term care institutions (Baltes et al., 1991).

Comparison of the various definitions of successful ageing

The five models of successful ageing described herein substantially differ from one another. While they are not necessarily exclusive to each other, they start from quite different views on successful ageing and rely on quite different normative building blocks in their efforts to define a good life at advanced age. So, what are the implications of choosing one of these model over another? To compare the five models, we use the following criteria:

- Age relevance: does the conception of successful ageing under analysis help spell out specific needs of older age groups?
- Inclusiveness: is the full range of older adults included in the conception of successful ageing or are some groups and/or subpopulations excluded from it?
- Locus of responsibility: is the model framed mostly individualistically or is there a role for society in taking responsibility for successful ageing?
- Normativity: does it include explicit statements on what norms and standards should drive successful ageing?
- Measurability: does the model provide clear strategies on how to operationalize and assess successful ageing at empirical level?

The result of our comparison can be found in Table 3.1. As can be seen, the five models differ starkly in terms of how they spell out specific needs of old age. Only the eudaimonic model specifies age-related challenges and developmental tasks. However, capability and care ethics-based models acknowledge the age-related progressive need for supportive structures. Both the pragmatic and hedonic models are age blind: being healthy and happy is relevant not only in old age, but throughout one's life course. The definitions also differ in scope and inclusiveness: while the capability- and care-related definitions explicitly include older individuals suffering impairments and in need of care, hedonic and eudaimonic definitions consider such groups at best

Table 3.1. Comparison of five models of successful ageing: pragmatic, hedonic, eudaimonic, capability, and care ethics-based models

	Pragmatic model	Hedonic model	Eudaimonic model	Capability-related model	Care ethics-based model
Age relevance	Low. Disease avoidance and functional health of relevance throughout life.	Low. Happiness and life satisfaction of relevance throughout life.	High. Developmental tasks are age-specific (e.g. wisdom in old age).	Medium. Structures enabling individuals to be and do what they value is relevant throughout life, although its relevance increases with age.	Medium. Providing support for someone's safety, health, and welfare is relevant throughout life, but its relevance increases with age.
Inclusiveness	Low. Older people with illness and disabilities are excluded.	High. Pursuit of happiness and life satisfaction open to all older people.	High. All older people have developmental tasks to deal with.	High. Depending on individual competence and goals, suitable opportunity structures should be available to all older people.	High. Supportive arrangements for one's safety, health, and welfare should be available to all older people.
Normativity	High. According to the model, health and fitness are prescriptive norms for successful ageing.	Medium. Being happy and satisfied is the prescriptive norm for successful ageing.	High. There are prescriptive norms regarding coping with developmental tasks for successful ageing.	Low. Successful ageing is based on individuals' values and competencies.	High. Successful ageing depends on care which is suitable for individual needs.

(Continued)

Table 3.1. *Continued*

	Pragmatic model	Hedonic model	Eudaimonic model	Capability-related model	Care ethics-based model
Locus of responsibility	Individual. Staying in good health until old age is mainly the responsibility of the individual, but external factors can be of help.	Individual. Happiness and life satisfaction is mainly the responsibility of the individual, but external factors can be of help.	Individual. Personal growth lies solely in the hand of the individual.	Society. Providing a diversity of opportunity structures for diverse goals and competencies is society's responsibility.	Society. Providing a system of high quality long-term care and support is society's responsibility.
Measurability	High. The outcomes of successful ageing (health and fitness) are easy to measure. Many validated measurement instruments available.	High. The outcomes of successful ageing (happiness and life satisfaction) are easy to measure. Many validated measurement instruments available.	Medium. The outcomes of successful ageing (solution of age-related developmental tasks) are not easy to measure. Few validated measurement instruments.	Low. Due to highly diverse constellations of goals, competence, and opportunity structure, measurement of successful ageing hardly possible.	Medium. Successful ageing as high-quality care (interaction between carer and person care for) is not easy to measure. Few validated measurement instruments.

implicitly, while the pragmatic definition flatly excludes this group entirely, treating such people as unsuccessful agers. While pragmatic, eudaimonic, and care-related definitions of successful ageing have a clear normative basis in how they assess outcomes as successful ageing (in terms of continued good health and active engagement, ability to cope sustainably with developmental tasks, or the existence of a supportive relationship between care recipient and caregiver), the hedonic and capability definitions appeal to less normative outcomes (looking at such variables as satisfaction with one's own life or goals achieved). In the pragmatic, hedonic, and eudaimonic models, responsibility for successful ageing rests on the shoulders of the individual, with wider society playing only a supporting role in the background. In the capability-related and care ethics-based models, society plays a much more important role. Within these two approaches, successful ageing seems impossible without tapping societal resources. Finally, turning to the issue of measurability, hedonic and pragmatic definitions lend themselves to fairly straightforward measurement procedures, while established procedures for measuring the 'success' of eudaimonic, capability- and care-related definitions are less clear and subject to ongoing methodological debates.

We close this chapter with a quote from Robert Havighurst: 'In gerontology it will probably be useful to use several different measures of successful ageing, always being explicit about their relations to operational definitions of successful ageing. In this way we are likely to learn more than if we limit ourselves to one theory and one definition of successful ageing, with its appropriate measure' (Havighurst, 1961, p.12). On that note, we now turn to the question of what processes and strategies we might use to help to bring about successful ageing, in strategies with targets ranging from the micro (individual responsibility) to the macro level (societal responsibility).

PART II

STRATEGIES FOR
SUCCESSFUL AGEING

From the micro to the macro level

4

Individual strategies
for successful ageing

The models of successful ageing detailed in the previous chapter describe endpoints or outcomes of positive development over the course of one's life. If one were to summarize each model in the form of a brief appeal or recommendation on how to accomplish successful ageing, one might make the following statements:

- be fit (the pragmatic model);
- be happy (the hedonic model);
- be wise (the eudaimonic model);
- be provided with the appropriate opportunity structures to pursue your goals (the capability-related model);
- be provided with the support to satisfy your needs (the care ethics-based model).

This exercise makes it clear that the various models of successful ageing each call for very different strategies and interventions in any effort to reach the outcomes defined for each of them. The first three models—the pragmatic, hedonic, and eudaimonic models—address the individual striving to reach their desired endpoints: to be fit, to be happy, or to be wise, respectively. External factors may be in place to support the individual's effort to age successfully, but the primary responsibility for successful ageing lies mainly in the hands of the individual.

The capability-related model and the care ethics-based model, however, encompass factors beyond the realm of the individual: that of being provided with opportunity structures or support. Both models describe successful ageing as being contextual in nature. By definition, the outcomes of efforts to age successfully are the result of the combined efforts of the individual and the context in which they are living. According to both models, therefore, responsibility for successful ageing is not simply a matter for the individual, but one that also rests on environmental actors. Strategies for successful ageing should aim to intervene on the interaction between the individual and the living situation in which that individual is embedded.

In this and the chapters to follow, we argue that strategies for successful ageing must chime well with the above-described models, but different strategies may resonate with different models. In this chapter we discuss strategies for successful ageing at the individual level. Then, in Chapter 5, we go on to focus on physical–spatial contexts and, in Chapter 6, on care contexts. Finally, we tackle the question of how policies of the welfare state may be harnessed to promote successful ageing (Chapter 7).

Pragmatic model strategies

Leading a healthy lifestyle—engaging in physical activity, eating healthily, and avoiding harmful substances—provides the main strategy for maintaining good health up into old age. Physical activity seems to be looked upon as an especially universal remedy against the perils of old age (Daskalopoulou et al., 2017). There is now robust evidence that physical activity can lead to 'reduced cardiometabolic risk, reduced risk of falls, improved cognitive function and functional capacity, and reduced risk of depression, anxiety, and dementia' (Bauman et al., 2016, p. S268). Eating healthy (Lorenzo-López et al., 2017) and avoiding harmful substances such as nicotine (Bosnes et al., 2019) also makes a significant preventative contribution to good health in old age. In addition, the willingness to engage oneself actively in volunteer work is not simply a consequence of enjoying good health, but actually produces a positive feedback loop in one's health (Hinterlong et al., 2007; Pillemer et al., 2010). The implications are straightforward: encouraging individuals, from youth into old age, to pursue a healthy lifestyle, to do volunteer work, and to engage actively in society will surely bring about successful ageing.

However, it might be that this vision turns out to be somewhat overoptimistic. Epidemiological data show that the chronic diseases and geriatric syndromes, including coronary heart disease, chronic obstructive pulmonary disease, cancer, and Alzheimer's disease, for instance, as well as general frailty and sarcopenia (Fortin et al., 2010), all increase with age. Hence, it would appear highly unlikely that health promotion and prevention measures will ever have the capacity to prevent age-related diseases entirely. Reflecting, in particular, on Rowe and Kahn's model of successful ageing, one might therefore well ask the question whether it is at all possible to maintain 'physical and cognitive functioning' and 'engagement in social and productive activities' even in the face of increasingly debilitating age-related diseases and disability (see also Chapters 5 and 6). A variety of theories of developmental regulation have been conceived in order to address this issue. One of the best-known approaches in this field is a model referred to as 'selective optimization with compensation' (Baltes & Baltes, 1990b). According to this account, older people facing age-related losses adopt three approaches in their efforts to preserve their autonomy and mastery of their lives: selecting manageable goals; optimizing their still uncompromised competencies; and using compensatory measures to achieve those goals. In other words, the combination of flexibility in adjusting one's goals and the tenacious pursuit of those goals provide the preconditions for successful ageing in the face of age-related obstacles (Brandtstädter & Renner, 1990). In a similar vein, other scholars rely on concepts referred to as 'primary control' (investing competence and effort) and 'secondary control' (changing aspirations and aims in life (Heckhausen & Buchmann, 2019; Heckhausen & Schulz, 1993)). Coping with age-related losses through managing resources and orchestrating regulation processes allows older people to participate actively and productively in everyday life (Wurm & Tesch-Römer, 2021). Hence, the pragmatic model of successful ageing remains applicable even if and when one's health becomes compromised in old age (Gignac et al., 2000).

Hedonic model strategies

With its focus on subjective well-being, the hedonic model shares one particular challenge with its pragmatic counterpart: how can one protect one's life satisfaction in the face of the irretrievable losses that inevitably come with advancing age? Achieving one's goals and maintaining one's capacities contributes positively to a person's life satisfaction, just as failing to do so leads to dissatisfaction and dysthymia. As one advances in age, increasing numbers of goals are permanently put out of reach by the onset of irreversible age-related losses. Although it seems logical to expect subjective life satisfaction to decline with age, empirical studies show surprising evidence of what is often referred to as the already referred to life satisfaction paradox: satisfaction with one's life tends to remain quite high until very late in life (e.g. Gatz & Zarit, 1999; McAdams et al., 2012).

In order to explain the paradox, one may yet again appeal to strategies involving the regulation of one's individual development, this time focusing not on agency, but rather on subjective well-being. When goals become permanently blocked—something that often happens in old age—continuing to pursue such goals ceases to be an adaptive strategy. In such situations, a pattern of flexible goal adjustment tends to take on an increasingly central role in the life strategies of older people. The practices of substituting goals—i.e. giving up unrealistic aims and choosing new ones—and of lowering one's expectations in relation to existing goals together open up a path to maintaining one's life satisfaction well into old age (Brandtstädter, 2009; Brandtstädter & Renner, 1990; compare, however, Tesch-Römer, 2005). Such practices can remain effective even until the end of life. Although the 'distance-to-death' research has observed a decline in life satisfaction in the situation of impending death (Gerstorf et al., 2008), yet even in this very last phase of life the adoption of secondary control strategies help to maintain one's well-being by focusing on those life domains that suffer the least impairment—such as social integration, for instance (Gerstorf et al., 2016).

However, a word of caution. Concentrating on the effort to achieve the best possible subjective well-being can come at a cost. Decisions by ageing individuals to avoid experiences they assess as negative in the short run can be harmful to their overall well-being. Medical examinations, for example, can cause anxiety but may turn out to be positive in the long run (Löckenhoff & Carstensen, 2004). Yet engaging in processes of developmental regulation to readjust one's life goals can make the pursuit of happiness—i.e. successful ageing as defined in hedonic terms—possible right up until the end of one's life.

Eudaimonic model strategies

How do we achieve wisdom as we grow old? What makes people accept their own life choices, banish regret, reject despair, and achieve a sense of integrity for themselves? According to Erikson's theory of psychosocial development and, as shown in the previous sections, being able to reflect on one's life is a precondition for the capacity to resolve of the psychosocial crises that tend to arise at the end of life, which prominently include the crisis that so often arises between ego integrity and despair (Erikson, 1982). Regardless of the intuitive appeal of the eudaimonic model of successful ageing, it seems difficult to disentangle its processes from its possible outcomes. The idea of reaching a 'dynamic balance of opposites' can be looked upon either as the result of coping successfully with a psychosocial crisis or as the coping strategy itself (Kivnick & Wells, 2014).

One might cautiously assert that the eudaimonic pathway can be identified as efforts to cope with the essential challenges of old age—hence achieving ego integrity and wisdom, while fending off despair. A number of strategies have been described in the literature: reminiscence (i.e. remembering and reflecting upon events and experiences from one's past (Pasupathi & Carstensen, 2003; Staudinger, 2001), as well as making the shift from the executive and outward-oriented processes that tend to feature during middle adulthood to the more inward processes of old age (Ryff, 1982). However, all of these strategies may have their downsides. The process of reminiscence, for instance, must be handled with care. It is important to keep a balance between positive and negative memories when recalling one's life, as focusing solely on negative events ('bitterness revival') can become a cause of sorrow and despair (Webster, 1993). Yet reminiscence, properly guided, can help to use one's memories, such as in reminiscence therapy to achieve positive outcomes (Butler, 1968). Studies indicate that reminiscence therapy can reinforce feelings of lifetime accomplishment and reduce levels of depression (Chiang et al., 2010).

Another pathway toward achieving an ego integrity-friendly state of mind in old age can be found in gerotranscendence theory (Tornstam, 2005). Tornstam argues that the major challenge of late life is the task of making a transition from a materialistic and rationalistic perspective to a more cosmic and transcendent view of life. This transition involves a redefinition of time, place, life, and death, and may result in the person practising a sort of solitary meditation and acquiring the ability to tap 'transcendental sources of happiness' (Tornstam, 2005, p. 59). These changes may be echoed, for example, in a new experience of nature, one that evokes a feeling of being one with the universe. As one participant in Tornstam's studies put it, 'I see trees, buds, and I see it blossom, and I see how the leaves are coming—I see myself in the leaves' (Tornstam, 2005, p. 59). It should be noted, however, that empirical data in respect to the emergence of gerotranscendence are quite scanty and that practically no longitudinal data exist to support the idea and its successful ageing outcomes.

Finally, gerontological research on religiosity and spirituality deserves mentioning. Both phenomena point to a quest to find answers to some of the ultimate questions about life, on the meaning of one's existence, and on one's relationship to the sacred or transcendent. These answers that may (or may not) either arise from or lead to the emergence of religious rituals and formation of communities (Koenig et al., 2001). Evidence suggests that the use of spiritual and religious means to help one cope with life tends to increase with age, although there seem to be no complete and readily available explanations as to why this should be the case (Krause, 2006). One explanation might be that the generally positive attitude to the use of religion to help one cope with age reflects the fact that people generally become more involved in religion as they grow older. Another reason can be traced in the stressful factors that especially confront people in later life (e.g. serious disease and the death of loved ones). In the last phase of one's life, one is also often forced to face one's missed opportunities, mistakes, and the unfortunate events one has witnessed—all which must be seen as water under the bridge, as things that one can no longer do anything about. In reflecting on the past, each person needs to come to terms with their life just as they have lived it. Eudaimonic strategies for successful ageing may help to create a coherent narrative of one's own biography. Still, it seems unlikely that there is any direct link between getting older and becoming wiser (Baltes & Staudinger, 2000).

Comparison of individual strategies for successful ageing

Despite the inherent differences between the goals of promoting health, regulating one's personal development and reconstructing a positive retrospective of one's life, some similarities are still detectible in these strategies. Firstly, they all put the responsibility for striving to age successfully firmly in the hands of the individual. Secondly, an individual's strategies for successful ageing require them to possess the adaptive resources they need to realign the vision of their present or former selves. Substituting one's goals and reconstructing one's biography require an ability on the part of the individual to hold a self-image that is both coherent and yet malleable. Thirdly, there may be external resources available to support the individual in their effort to achieve successful ageing. With these insights in mind, we can now go on to look at the role played by a person's surrounding contexts in fostering or hindering successful ageing.

5

Physical–spatial–technological environments and successful ageing

The eminent relevance of the physical, spatial, and technological environment in the effort to achieve successful ageing has already been mentioned earlier in this book, noting that the capability-related and the care ethics-based models put a greater emphasis on environmental factors than do the pragmatic, hedonic and eudaimonic models. In this chapter we argue that one's physical, spatial, and technological environments are very relevant to successful ageing both in a conceptual and in a practical sense. Conceptually, we believe that effort towards ageing successfully cannot be discussed separately from the various external forces that serve as constraining or enhancing influences on that effort. From a practical point of view, interventions aimed at improving one's environment become increasingly relevant as an individual's resources and reserve capacities dwindle. Hence, interventions aimed at optimizing environments (e.g. in housing, the features of a neighbourhood, or public transport) have the capacity to enhance the potential available or successful ageing.

Theoretical conceptions of environmental contexts

Physical–spatial contexts shape our development throughout our lives. The physical–spatial environment encompasses a broad range of elements, including the built environment that provides housing and such neighbourhood facilities as local shops, recreational areas, and access to public transport, and also involves such matters as traffic volumes, air pollution, and crime. Wider geography, such as local authority areas and the features available in them also have the power to shape the lives of older people (Wahl & Gerstorf, 2018). Finally, access to and use of technology—both within and outside the home—also forms part of the set of environmental contexts within which ageing takes place.

The field of environmental gerontology (Lawton & Nahemow, 1973; Wahl et al., 2012) strives to understand the role of the physical–spatial environment in maintaining and improving the autonomy, well-being, and health of older people. One of the key propositions of environmental gerontology is that older people are particularly affected by their physical–spatial environment, and that their capacity for personal development can be either enhanced or constrained by environmental factors. Two examples might serve to clarify this point: an older person with dementia may no longer be able to navigate about their neighbourhood, but may find their way around in a well-designed housing arrangement designed to improve orientation for its cognitively impaired residents. In contrast, an older individual with difficulties in getting about on foot living in an apartment on an upper floor without a lift is likely to be constrained in their enjoyment of outdoor activities. Three conceptual frameworks relating to physical–spatial environments can be identified as relevant to the discourse on successful ageing: (1) personal environmental docility vs proactivity; (2) person–environment goodness vs badness of fit; and (3) one's sense of environmental belonging vs environmental disconnect.

Personal environmental docility versus proactivity

An idea often referred to as the environmental docility hypothesis contends that the fewer resources a person has at their disposal and the lower their level of competence, the greater the impact environmental factors is likely to have on their quality of life (Lawton & Simon, 1968). One consequence of this is that the physical–spatial features of an environment tend to affect individual outcomes more radically at low levels of competency and resources than they do at higher levels. However, growing older successfully is not simply an issue of seeing older people as 'suffering' from environmental docility, looking upon older adults as mere pawns in the interplay of what are often labelled environmental pressures (Lawton & Nahemow, 1973). The concept of proactivity takes in the vision of ageing individuals as active and goal-directed shapers of their environments (Lawton, 1989). The concept of proactivity overlaps generously with the notion of person–environment agency as an umbrella term for one's capacity to exert self-efficacy in pursuit of the goal of adapting and optimizing one's physical–spatial environment to one's needs (Wahl et al., 2012).

Fit and lack of fit of the person–environment system

As people age, a gap more often than not develops in the fit between the ageing person's competence and their environment. The most widely held understanding of the notion of person–environment fit is driven by objective characteristics (i.e. by a significant gap that opens out between an ageing person's functional competencies and the physical–spatial situations in which that person lives) (Iwarsson, 2004). The main assumption behind this concept is that the objective characteristics of the physical–spatial environment do not *per se* constitute a risk, but only become a risk once one's functional limitations begin to mean that one no longer has the capacity to deal with and compensate for those characteristics in the given context. The model based on person–environment fit thus predicts that if one's personal characteristics do not suit the given physical–spatial environment, the result will be a loss of autonomy, lower levels of well-being, and higher levels of depression. Such issues may be particularly difficult for vulnerable older people. For example, people suffering from dementia tend to be more sensitive to their surroundings and their dependency on the environment will increase as their illness develops. However, a dementia-friendly design, adapted to the needs and abilities of users, can provide support for the functional abilities of users and thus contribute to maintaining as good a fit as possible between person and environment (Marquardt et al., 2014).

Environmental belonging versus environmental disconnect

A sense of person–environment belonging means one's enjoyment of a positive attachment to one's physical–spatial environment and the creation of some level of place identity (Wahl et al., 2012). One of the strongest needs felt by humans is the need to form social attachments and to resist the dissolution of the bonds they have already formed (Baumeister & Leary, 1995). Translating this observation into the physical–spatial environment, a sense of belonging includes a high level of satisfaction with where one resides, positive socio-emotional perceptions of the physical–spatial location in which one lives, and a feeling of comfort (Oswald & Wahl, 2005). If such a cognitive–emotional attachment to place declines, or if it becomes impossible to construct in a new physical–spatial environment, the result may be what is referred to as person–environment disconnect. The experience that one's needs are no longer fulfilled by one's physical–spatial place may result in a feeling of alienation, of being lost, of being a stranger in one's own living arrangements.

Relevance of the environment for models of successful ageing

Physical–spatial environments can have great relevance to models for successful ageing. Table 5.1 illustrates some possible links between conceptual frameworks in connection with physical–spatial environments and models of successful ageing. As the table depicts, the challenges of docility/agency and person–environment fit take on particular importance within the pragmatic, capability, and care ethics models. In contrast, the hedonic and eudaimonic models predominantly reveal an affinity between the environmental belonging/disconnect challenge, on the one hand, and physical–spatial environments, on the other. The fact that the vulnerable section of the older population is particularly targeted by the care ethics model of successful ageing would suggest that the belonging/disconnect challenge may also be expected to have a good deal of significance in that model, making it the only model of all the ones listed to require optimal spatial–physical environment solutions with respect to all three person–environment challenges.

Types of environmental contexts and successful ageing

Physical–spatial environment can be conceptualized on various levels. Housing conditions (both in private homes and in long-term care institutions), constitute the micro-level, one's neighbourhood and community the meso-level, and larger geographical units (such as municipalities and local government areas) combine a range of meso-level units. In addition, technology cuts across all these levels of analysis. In the following paragraphs we discuss selected categories of physical-spatial environments.

Housing

Remaining as long as possible in one's own private home is likely to be the preferred physical–spatial option for older adults all over the world, even though housing quality varies dramatically from country to country and

Table 5.1. Relevance of the environment for models of successful ageing

	Person–environment docility vs proactivity	Person–environment fit vs lack of fit	Person–environment belonging vs disconnect
Relevance for pragmatic model of successful ageing	Relevant: successful ageing implies practising person–environment proactivity and agency and avoiding person–environment docility	Relevant: person–environment fit is an important prerequisite for unfolding one's full potential for successful ageing	Less relevant
Relevance for hedonic model of successful ageing	Less relevant	Less relevant	Relevant: feeling satisfied with and experiencing comfort in one's physical–spatial environment forms part of successful ageing
Relevance for eudaimonic model of successful ageing	Less relevant	Less relevant	Relevant: a sense of cognitive–emotional place is important for creating meaning and purpose in life
Relevance for capability-related model of successful ageing	Relevant: capabilities can only be fully exploited in physical–spatial environments that foster proactivity and avoid docility	Relevant: optimal exploitation of one's capabilities is only possible where person–environment fit is optimal	Less relevant
Relevance for care ethics-based model of successful ageing	Relevant: for people in need of care, the physical–spatial environment can stimulate proactivity and attenuate environmental docility	Relevant: for people in need of support and care, appropriate housing and out-of-house environments can secure a good person–environment fit	Relevant: for people in need of care it is crucial to maximize one's sense of environmental belonging, even in high-level care environments such as long-term care institutions

from world region to world region. Empirical research demonstrates a strong association between high levels of housing-related agency, strong feelings of belonging, and a good person–environment fit to compensate for functional impairments, on the one hand, and such outcomes as positive affect, absence of depressive moods, and feelings of autonomy, on the other (Iwarsson et al., 2007; Oswald et al., 2007).

Institutional living

Nursing homes may serve as most fitting environments for significant subsections of the older adult population suffering multimorbidity, loss of functional capacities, and weak or overburdened social networks by providing effective compensation for lost competencies and facilitating activities and social interaction (Baltes et al., 1991). Still, the nursing home remains an ambivalent environment for successful ageing owing to the inherent threat it implies to one's ability to exert proactivity and agency, to one's sense of belonging, and to one's dignity. In an effort to produce a more homelike nursing home environment, all kinds of design and organizational improvements are being tested worldwide, but the evidence that such efforts can significantly enhance the quality of life of residents remains rather equivocal, particularly for those who suffer from dementia, and their capacity to improve work satisfaction among staff (Ausserhofer et al., 2016).

Neighbourhood

The importance of the physical–spatial neighbourhood environment still seems all too frequently underestimated in discussions on successful ageing (Wahl & Gerstorf, 2018). This neglect reveals itself as particularly unfortunate given the abundant evidence that has emerged out of gerontology and epidemiology to show that improved neighbourhood features are linked with better functional capacities (Wilkinson et al., 2017) and improved mental and physical health (Eibich et al., 2016), not to mention walking abilities (Mendes de Leon et al., 2009), among older people. Neighbourhood features such as street connectivity and walkability also have implications for community participation in general (Vaughan et al., 2016). Of note, where the quality of a neighbourhood is low, relocation to better-fitting places may seem an obvious solution. However, the strong cognitive–affective ties that older adults have to their homes and neighbourhoods after the decades they spent growing old in them, make it quite an effort for them to decide on which place is likely to provide the best support for their successful ageing. On top of that personal factor, the assessment that one's neighbourhood represents a physical–spatial environment of major importance in successful ageing is also closely linked to looking upon the communities as a key setting in the task of ageing well (Greenfield et al., 2019).

Municipalities and local authority areas

The role of the characteristics exhibited by municipalities and local authority areas in relation to successful ageing has been illustrated in a range of new data that have emerged from recent studies. For example, Gerstorf and colleagues reported that the characteristics of local authority areas can explain a substantial part of the variance in late-life well-being outcomes between individuals, similar to the effect on well-being typically accounted for by physical health (Gerstorf et al., 2010b). Similarly, in local authority areas equipped with more inpatient care facilities, more care staff per resident, and more administrative staff one finds much improved end-of-life well-being—a particularly important indicator for the very oldest adults (Vogel et al., 2018).

Technology

Under the heading of digital technology comes everything from assistive devices and robotics to new communication tools for use both within and outside one's home. This type of 'virtual or enhanced environment' technology has been increasingly catching the eye of researchers into successful ageing since turn of the millennium (Charness & Schaie, 2003; Lee & Riek, 2018; Rowe & Kahn, 2015). Technology can contribute to maintaining or enhancing the health of older individuals in various ways (Schulz et al., 2015). For example, there is now a wide variety of intelligent measuring or monitoring devices available in the healthcare field. Technology can also be used in the delivery of such interventions as remote behavioural treatment of depression and in helping patients to manage chronic disease. Researchers have recently reported on a positive initial assessment of a technology-based training programme for imparting everyday skills to older adults (Czaja et al., 2020). Technology may also be used to help people preserve their cognitive functioning through providing cognitive training opportunities (Kamin & Lang,

2020). Likely even more important, technology may be used to provide external 'cognitive compensation' when a person's cognitive performance has become impaired. However, the use of a technological device is adaptive only as long as the pay-offs in terms of released (cognitive) resources are greater than its handling costs (e.g. in terms of cognitive resources that one needs to invest (Lindenberger et al., 2008)). Finally, technology can take on a crucial role in counteracting social isolation and fostering social engagement among older adults (Czaja et al., 2018).

Physical–spatial environment's impact on successful ageing

To conclude this chapter, the frequently overlooked roles and impacts of the physical–spatial environment deserve more attention in discussions about models and potential actions for successful ageing. Taking physical–spatial environment into account also broadens the scope of potential interventions available to ensure or provide support for successful ageing. For example, home modifications and/or the systematic improvement of the physical–spatial housing environment may be seen as an important strategy to support successful ageing by helping to improve the functional capacity and safe mobility of older people within their own homes, as well as reinforcing their confidence that they can remain in their own home for as long as humanly possible (Wahl et al., 2009; Wahl & Gitlin, 2018). Digital technologies also have the potential to support successful ageing in a variety of ways. Given the growing need among a great many older adults to stay in their homes even after their care needs and physical/mental impairments have become substantial, one of the major challenges for successful ageing in the future will be how to equip private homes to fulfil care-related needs that are currently provided for the most part through institutional long-term care. This future task of supporting ageing *in situ* even where an individual has suffered a significant loss of competence is certainly likely to develop in close connection with digital technologies, smart home interventions, and robotic aids (Lee & Riek, 2018; Schulz et al., 2015).

6

Social bonds, care, and successful ageing

We do not live and grow old in isolation, but together with one another. Not only are we embedded in our physical environments (as detailed in Chapter 5), but also in the social network formed by our family, friends, and neighbours. These social bonds are a necessary precondition for successful self-development over the course of our lives. Childhood is the phase of human development in which one needs love, protection, guidance, and supervision from significant others to unfold one's full potential through making best of use of the various developmental areas available to one (Sameroff, 2009). Social bonds continue to exert central importance all through one's lifespan and include a wide variety of relationships in a multitude of domains from education and work to leisure activities and civic participation. Social relations are a key factor in ageing—as they are over the whole of one's life course—and ageing research has demonstrated the importance of social relations in achieving positive outcomes and avoiding loneliness in old age (Antonucci et al., 2014; Tesch-Römer & Huxhold, 2019). Nevertheless, advanced old age often brings with it losses in functional abilities and an increased need for support and help. We argue that social embeddedness—from informal support through to formal care situations—provides the key to understanding successful ageing, even in cases of extreme frailty and dependency on care.

It should be emphasized here that Rowe and Kahn (e.g. 1997) have already highlighted the key roles played by social relations and social support in successful ageing. Empirical research since then has confirmed and expanded our knowledge on the critical role played by social bonding in successful ageing (including, for instance, Antonucci et al., 2011; Rook, 2015). Longitudinal research on ageing couples has, for example, shown that the long-term development of health, cognitive performance, and well-being depends to a significant extent on the social phenomenon that any change affecting one life partner will tend to drive change in the other and vice versa (Hoppmann & Gerstorf, 2016). Similarly, research on 'interactive minds' (Staudinger & Baltes, 1996), collaborative cognition (Staudinger & Baltes, 1996), and intergenerational interchange (Kessler & Staudinger, 2007) has shown that older adults profit in terms of their cognitive functioning and a greater complexity in their emotional regulation ability from solving cognitive and other tasks in social contexts together with their partners, with other older adults and with adolescents. Concluding, Rowe and Kahn's (1997) third criterion for successful ageing—engagement with life—has meanwhile found empirical support and differentiation at various levels.

What has so far been missing from this discourse on successful ageing is the role that caring family members and professional caregivers can take on, particularly with respect to successful ageing in advanced old age, although the care ethics model represents an exception to this observation (see Chapter 3). For this reason, we discuss the role of care in successful ageing informed by the care ethics model. But, before doing so, we think it important to discuss the role played by morbidity, functional loss, and care in the process of growing old, and how that role is likely to become even more important in the decades to come.

Morbidity, functional loss, and care needs as a reality of old age

The irreversible losses of old age have the effect of restricting individual agency. Poor health and declining cognitive abilities can often undermine the efficiency and robustness of a person's self-regulation processes (Gerstorf & Ram, 2015; Wahl & Gerstorf, 2018). The very end of life—dying and death— can pose challenges to an individual's self-determination and dignity. There is reason to believe that (lifelong) preventative and health promotion efforts may bring with them antagonistic effects in both the short and the long term. While health promotion and prevention may improve health status in the earlier years of old age ('Third Age'), it may also have the effect of prolonging one's lifespan, and perhaps eventually lead to longer phases of ill health and frailty in late life ('Fourth Age', see Tesch-Römer & Wahl, 2017).

Early hopes of achieving an absolute compression of morbidity (i.e. a smaller number of years spent in ill health by each successive birth cohort; Fries, 1980) now look less well-founded than they used to (Crimmins et al., 2016). While life expectancy has grown steadily over the years, its rate of growth has slowed over the last decade (Crimmins, 2021). Although it is true that the relative share of healthy life expectancy within total life expectancy rose between 2000 and 2012, and that some evidence for compression of morbidity has been detected in the USA (Harper, 2014; Stallard, 2016), the evidence available at global level tends to suggest a relative increase in both healthy *and* unhealthy life expectancy. This can be seen in data from the Global Burden of Disease Study, which was based on 187 countries, comparing figures for 1990 against 2010 (Salomon et al., 2012; see also Beltrán-Sánchez et al., 2014; Crimmins & Beltrán-Sánchez, 2011; Crimmins et al., 2016). Social inequality also plays a role in this phenomenon (Crimmins, 2021): where compression of morbidity is actually occurring, it is closely connected with higher levels of educational attainment (Jagger et al., 2008), revealing that the path to low morbidity in the last phase of one's life is reserved for the better off (for the influence of social inequality on ageing, see also Dannefer, 2003; Ferraro & Shippee, 2009). Hence, it now seems high time to at least adjust, if not to abandon altogether, the 1980s vision of healthy ageing up to the end of life.

In the past, we have seen continuously increasing slices of healthy *and* unhealthy life expectancy, suggesting that it is increasingly likely for all of us to experience an ageing process involving a need for care. Yet successful ageing models that focus solely on preserving functional fitness and participation in society would seem to be restricted to the healthy phases in the second half of one's life and thus the 'Third Age'. From that perspective, the 'Fourth Age', now a steadily expanding portion of one's lifespan, would be excluded from the prospects of successful ageing. We argue, on the contrary, that successful ageing is possible even after multiple morbidity, functional loss, and cognitive impairment have begun to set in in old age, and that what it takes to achieve successful ageing under such conditions is adequate care.

Care and successful ageing

Central to care and caring are the social relations and social networks formed by the people caring for those in need of that care. Care ethics, the philosophical approach discussed in Chapter 3, is fundamentally based on social bonds. According to this approach, the act of caring consists of a set of interrelated activities between care giver and care receiver (Tronto, 2014). In our view, for ageing individuals in need of care and support, successful ageing should be seen as the outcome of a shared process between the caregiver and the care recipient in which the caregivers provide their care in an attentive, responsible, and competent manner, while the care receivers respond positively to these acts of support (Lachman, 2012).

Orem's nursing theory is based upon the idea that people have a 'need for self-care', i.e., that they would like to care for themselves (Orem & Taylor, 2011). However, individuals may vary in their self-care demands (owing to illness, disability, or frailty) and in terms of their self-care agency (owing to lack of resources or knowledge). When caring for a person, caregivers are required to use their (professional) competence and knowledge (nursing agency) to help individuals in their efforts to fulfil their self-care needs. Where self-reliance and autonomy come under threat—in old age, because of increasing multiple morbidity, disability, and frailty—care is there to support the older person in their efforts to retain their autonomy.

In *Roy's adaptation model of nursing* the focus shifts from personal needs to the notion of adaptation. Individuals are seen as biopsychosocial entities who interact systematically with their physical and social environment (Roy, 2011). The goal of this interaction with one's environment is to achieve adaptation in four different modes: physiological–physical, self-concept, role function, and interdependence. Nursing interventions are necessary when disturbances such as illness or disability affect the system as defined by the individual embedded in the environment. The goal of nursing is to promote adaptation in these four modes, contributing to one's health and one's quality of life, and helping one to die with dignity.

One of the earliest nursing theories, *Peplau's interpersonal relationship theory*, emphasizes the relationship between caregiver and care recipient as the basis for nursing practice (Peplau, 1997). Nursing practice must strive to achieve learning experiences in the interaction between caregiver and care recipient. In respect of old age, the appeal of this theory lies in the interactive nature of the care process; care provider and care recipient interact reciprocally within the process described by the theory to reach joint decisions.

Finally, *Paterson and Zderad's humanistic nursing theory* emerged from the notion that people express their needs in verbal and non-verbal requests or 'calls' concerning a health-related issue (Paterson & Zderad, 1976; Silva, 2013). In perceiving, understanding, and responding to these calls, the caregiver must communicate with the care recipient in order to understand, value, and respect the person's situation. In this communication process, the caregiver should always be aware of him or herself and of the client as unique persons. Central to this position is an understanding of the person's perspective, identity, and needs. Hence, nursing is not so much about restoring lost health as a process of mutual understanding and a search for meaning right up until the end of life.

Taking the essence of these theories together as they relate to successful ageing in situations where there is a need for care, we arrive at the following conclusions: all four models have in common that imagining successful ageing with concentrated care needs must rely on interactive processes with professional or informal care providers and with other elements of the context in which the cared-for individuals live, such as their physical home environment and the assistive technology that may be available to them. The effort to achieve successful ageing while confronting one's frailty and facing major functional loss is a human condition that fundamentally calls out for a support process. Such support cannot eliminate or even reduce the resource loss that the ageing process has produced, particularly not in a situation of chronic disease and functional impairment—a circumstance typical of advanced old age. However, high-quality support in caring also involves enhancing the person's remaining capacity for autonomy and facilitating as far as possible the attainment of those of their life goals still within reach, thus allowing their personal growth as a realistic possibility.

End-of-life care as a particular challenge for successful ageing

Death and dying represent a major facet of care in old age—whether in home health care, in acute hospital care, or in long-term care institutions. When we argue that successful ageing is possible even for old adults with extensive care needs, a question then logically arises as to whether it could make sense to speak of 'successful dying'. Yet matters of dying and death are not a much favoured theme for theorists and empirical researchers in the successful ageing landscape. In a paper entitled 'New frontiers in the future of ageing: from successful ageing of the young old to the dilemmas of the Fourth Age', Paul Baltes and Jacqui Smith make clear even in the title of their work that the Fourth Age represents a major threat to successful ageing—and to dying with dignity, in particular (Baltes & Smith, 2003). In the already annotated excellent collection of papers published in the special issues on successful ageing by *The Gerontologist* (2015) and the *Journal of Gerontology* (2017), almost nothing can be found on the topic of death and dying. The scholars that do address death and dying in the context of successful ageing are rare exceptions (one example would be Wong, 1989).

And yet the notion of successful dying and its proximity to the concept of a 'good death' (Cottrell & Duggleby, 2016; Meier et al., 2016), has attracted considerable attention in recent years. In a review on existing ideas about what it means to have a successful and good death, three themes stood out: 'preferences for dying process', 'pain-free status', and 'emotional well-being' (Meier et al., 2016). Note that the 'preferences for dying process' category included the following subthemes: the death scene (how, who, where, and when), dying during sleep, and preparation for death (e.g. advance directives/living will and funeral arrangements). Hugely important factors in a 'good death' include the place of and the social support provided during the process of dying. A study by Dasch et al. (2015) provides evidence on trends in Germany. The findings show that a clear majority of all deaths in Germany occurred in 2015 in acute hospitals (54 per cent), followed by deaths in private households (25 per cent), and in nursing homes (15 per cent). About four per cent died in hospices or palliative units, with the remaining deaths occurring elsewhere. Being older than 80 years of age clearly increases one's likelihood of dying in an acute hospital or nursing home but reduces one's chances of dying at home. Differences between countries are, however, large. In the USA, for instance, numbers dying at home surpassed the figures for dying in an acute hospital in 2019 (Cross & Warraich, 2019). It is noteworthy that the majority declare a preference for dying either at home or in a hospice (Gomes et al., 2011), but will not see that final wish satisfied (Dixon et al., 2019). A study in four European countries also showed that patients' preferred place of death was often unknown to the general practitioners, i.e. older adults' most direct health authority, suggesting widespread ignorance of this as an issue among major medical institutions (De Roo et al., 2014). This brief overview demonstrates the need to apply the ideas of successful ageing to the challenges of end-of-life care: protecting a dying person's autonomy, dignity, and well-being, while providing caring forms an essential ingredient in successful ageing (Gott & Ingleton, 2011; Jeong et al., 2010).

Need for a qualitative turn in the discourse on successful ageing

We have argued in this chapter that the effort to achieve successful ageing needs to consider social bonds (as we argued in Chapter 5). This insight has fundamental consequences for successful ageing. We posit that models of successful ageing in addition to the ones based purely and simply on the perspective of individual agency are needed (such as Rowe and Kahn's model, for example). Successful ageing models have to acknowledge the critical importance of collective support during the phases of life in which a person begins to require care, models that pursue the aim of supporting that person's personal dignity, quality of life, and self-determined agency.

Hence, we need to achieve a qualitative turn in the discourse on successful ageing, away from an exclusive focus on the striving for agency and towards accepting weakness and working to provide adequate support and care. Such a change in the direction of our view becomes necessary because in the future a great many life-course trajectories can be expected to contain phases of restricted functional ability and impaired cognitive capacity. One way of illustrating the point graphically (see Fig. 6.1) would be to plot four different trajectories for functional ability. As the figure shows, levels of functional ability begin to diverge as early as in young adulthood, possibly as a result of social inequality. Each of the four trajectories shown differ from all the others: while individual A shows a steady level of functional ability well into old age, for individuals B and D that level begins to decline in midlife, and C's functional ability actually experiences a boost in later life. Nevertheless, all four trajectories end up crossing a functional threshold at some stage or other. We define this functional threshold as the level at which one's agency as exerted in one's earlier life becomes increasingly maladaptive due to loss of resources, and at which support accordingly begins to become adaptive. Note that life duration differs markedly between the four hypothetical lifetimes: logically enough, in order to be in a position to age successfully, any

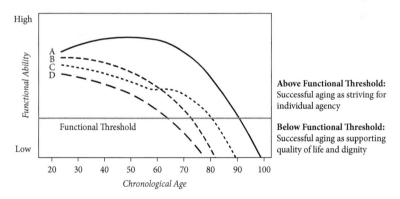

Fig. 6.1. Changes in importance of criteria for successful ageing depending on being above or below a functional threshold (modified after Hertzog et al., 2009).

person first needs to remain healthy for long enough to grow old in the first place (Dugravot et al., 2020).

Furthermore, we would assert that reprioritizing the fundamental criteria for successful ageing depending on whether one is above or below the functional threshold should be seen as requirement in the effort to achieve a qualitative shift in the criteria one needs to apply to be in a position to assess how successfully a person is ageing. What we have in mind, in other words, is a *gestalt* switch by which models of successful ageing should drastically and holistically transform the value system they apply as soon as ageing the relevant individual crosses their personal functional threshold. In order to be able to consider the idea of successful ageing among frail people suffering multiple morbidities seriously, we may need to follow new directions in how we construct our theory in gerontology, abandoning the widespread dichotomy that distinguishes between a 'world of successful ageing' and a 'world of care in old age'. It may even be that extending the significance of the concept of successful ageing to include older adults in need of care could help in softening this schismatic dividing line. Employing the concept of successful ageing as an important category in caring contexts may assist processes of meaning creation even in extreme life situations and may motivate one to make the best of use possible out of remaining reserve capacities at the level of the care recipient. However, support and care is not exclusively the task of care networks and care institutions. We also have to consider the societal conditions that provide the ground upon which the different pathways of successful ageing lie. This consideration of various macro-level factors remains a missing piece in the flow of our argument: one that we shall address in the next chapter.

7

Social inequality, the welfare state, and successful ageing

The task of re-engineering societal institutions is the bold vision behind Rowe and Kahn's (2015) call for an expansion of the pragmatic concept of successful ageing. Their thesis recommends that social policies be modified to better facilitate the health and active participation in society of older people. This would not only shape individual ageing trajectories in a positive direction, but would also help societies deal with the opportunities and problems exhibited by ageing demographics. We agree that the welfare state and social policies can play a role in achieving successful ageing. However, we consider it necessary to account for the overall function of the modern welfare state: to intervene in matters of societal inequality by applying policies on education, health, housing, social benefits, and social insurance (Eikemo & Bambra, 2008; Esping-Andersen, 1990). Before discussing the role of welfare state policies in successful ageing by focusing not simply on the pragmatic approach, but also on the hedonic, eudaimonic, capability-related, and care ethics-based models, we must first address the challenges that social inequality poses for successful ageing.

Social inequality as a basic challenge to successful ageing

Differences between individuals permeate our life courses from conception to death. While the concept of 'diversity' refers to horizontal differences between individuals, for example in relation to interests or lifestyles, the concept of 'inequality' points to vertical differences between individuals in connection with unevenly distributed access to goods and resources of value, such as education, prestige, income, and wealth. The disposal of valued resources draws the line between those who have and those who have not. Depending on one's access to resources, pathways through life may open or close up, with substantial effects on life outcomes (O'Rand, 2016). Empirical evidence, including studies focusing on successful ageing as an outcome, shows that unfavourable childhood conditions exert a harmful influence on individuals' chances for successful ageing, i.e. one's chances of avoiding any major illness or disability in the activities of one's daily life and of enjoying high-level cognitive functioning and of being actively engaged (Brandt et al., 2012; Ferraro et al., 2016).

Inequality-related differences between individuals may increase over one's life, owing to the accumulation of advantages or disadvantages, resulting in extensive and increasing disparities in middle adulthood and old age favouring people with greater resources (Dannefer, 2003; Ferraro et al., 2016; House et al., 2005). Although there is ongoing discussion about whether the impact of social inequality begins to diminish in very old age (Britton et al., 2008; Herd, 2006; Hu et al., 2020), it has been clearly established that people of lower socio-economic status tend, on average, to have a shorter lifespan than people higher up the ladder and that the former have a lower probability of living up into old age (Lewer et al., 2020). Even taking premature mortality into account, inequality gradients in terms of health, as well as other outcomes, persist right through adulthood and into old age, hampering the chances of ageing successfully among those of us with more modest resources (Ferraro et al., 2017; Hank, 2011).

Inequality is important not only at a micro level (i.e. in terms of individual access to resources), but it also plays out at the meso and macro levels. Differences between communities—a meso-level concept concerned with such geographical and administrative contexts as neighbourhoods, villages, local authority areas, and municipalities—also have a clear relationship with the health and well-being of older people (Greenfield et al., 2019). Neighbourhood features have a link to the functional status in older adults (Wilkinson et al., 2017), as well as their mental health (Wilson-Genderson & Pruchno, 2013), health behaviour (Schüz et al., 2014), physical health (Eibich et al., 2016), and walking ability (Mendes de Leon et al., 2009). Thus, the meso-level characteristics of the context in which one is living may alleviate (or exacerbate) inequality on an individual level, so that people living in more fortunate environments are more likely to age successfully.

In addition, macro-level structures and processes also play a role. Educational systems, vocational pathways, and social policies have the capacity to reinforce or alleviate inequality within a society. Such macro-level structures clearly influence an individual's life course and the opportunities they enjoy for successful ageing (Stowe & Cooney, 2015). Longevity is greater in more affluent societies; the greatest improvements in life expectancy in the past decades have occurred (at least in Europe) among the socio-economically advantaged and the smallest are found among the more disadvantaged countries (Leon, 2011). Such improvements are probably due to better living conditions, although they also have to do with more effective social security and healthcare systems. However, the amount of wealth in a society is not the only macro-factor that influences growing old and longevity: the extent of inequality within societies also plays a role. It has been shown that intercountry differences in life expectancy are related to differences in income equality, leading to the conclusion that societal inequality in a society has a negative impact on health outcomes not just for the disadvantaged, but for all members of that society (Banks et al., 2009; Wilkinson, 1996). More specifically, and appealing to Rowe and Kahn's pragmatic definition of successful ageing (Rowe & Kahn, 1997), empirical evidence suggests that lower levels of societal income inequality are associated with a greater probability of successful ageing—for all older members of a population (Brandt et al., 2012). Similarly, it has been argued on the basis of the eudaimonic model that unequal societies may compromise the potential for eudaimonic well-being of the less privileged (Ryff, 2017).

Gender and successful ageing

A central dimension of diversity and inequality concerns gender: the multifaceted differences between women and men that evolve over the life course. In many societies the average living situation of women is disadvantaged compared to that of men, and opportunity structures are unequally distributed between genders (UNDP, 2020, p. 361; cf. Dilli et al., 2019; Permanyer, 2013). Gender equality (or inequality) on a societal level has a variety of facets and includes, among others, gender specific opportunity structures (like gender differences in labour market participation), access to resources (like gender differences in average income), or power structures (like gender differences in parliamentary representation).

Gender differences in opportunity structures and action resources should affect also the opportunities for successful ageing. Interestingly, gender (and other aspects of diversity and inequality) has not played a prominent role in the development of Rowe and Kahn's pragmatic model of successful ageing. Rowe and Kahn (1997) mention gender only twice, and in a solely technical context, not a theoretical perspective. Empirical studies on gender differences show mixed findings which are highly dependent on definitions of successful ageing and covariates used in statistical analyses (Depp & Jeste,

2006). In respect to Rowe and Kahn's pragmatic model of successful ageing, it seems that women are less likely to age successfully than men (Hank, 2011; see, however, McLaughlin et al., 2010).

In terms of the hedonic model of successful ageing, Pinquart and Sörensen (2001) found in their meta-analysis significantly lower hedonic well-being for women. Gender differences in hedonic well-being are tied to the central aspect of the living situation of men and women: widowhood, health, and socio-economic status. Controlling for differences in respect of these contextual variables reduces the size of the differences between men and women, but the remaining gender gap is still significant (Pinquart & Sörensen, 2001). This trend is valid up to the present time worldwide, although the gap between women and men varies between countries (Carmel, 2019). In a comparative perspective, it has been shown that gender inequality on the societal level increases the gender gap in subjective quality of life (Tesch-Römer et al., 2008). Of note, the eudaimonic successful ageing model comes up with a quite different view of gender differences. The only consistent difference was found with respect to the dimension 'Social Relations with Others', which was higher in women, and some evidence also indicated 'Personal Growth' as being higher in older women. No differences were observed in the remaining dimensions (Ryff & Keyes, 1995).

The capability model and the care ethics model address the topic of gender from another perspective. The capability model considers different types of inequalities and argues that opportunity structures have to be improved in order to compensate for disadvantages on the individual level. Hence, gender differences in income, health, and subjective well-being are not taken as results of successful ageing, but as a starting point to enable both women and men to pursue goals they value. Similarly, the care ethics model of successful ageing comes with a close affinity to gender issues. Most individuals cared for are women, and the majority of caregivers, both in formal and informal contexts, are female. Comparing female and male caregivers shows that females experience more caregiving stress than men (Swinkels et al., 2019). Hence, men have to be encouraged to take on care responsibilities. In the last few years, men have started, although at a low level, to take over family care roles more often, for example for their wives with dementia (Hellström et al., 2017).

In the debate on critical gerontology the construct of gender gained visibility in the 1990s (e.g. Calasanti & Slevin, 2001) and has remained high on the agenda since then. A central argument in this debate refers to the concept of gender as a 'personal characteristic'. As Calasanti and King (2020) argue, it is problematic to analyse gender differences—similar to race and socioeconomic inequalities—without linkage to societal structures and the influences of welfare states. In the next section, we take up this argument and discuss the role of the welfare state in successful ageing.

Welfare state policies and successful ageing

When one considers diversity and inequality in a population, welfare states reveal themselves as central actors in shaping requirements for successful ageing. Hence, our next step is to discuss how policies might be applied to further successful ageing (for an in-depth discussion, see Tesch-Römer, 2020). Our key argument, following what has already been said, is that the particular design of social policy one chooses will depend on what conceptions of successful ageing one adopts and, accordingly, what outcomes one aims for. Depending on those choices, one could prioritize fitness, happiness, wisdom, autonomous capacity, or high-quality care. In other words, there is no single social policy for successful ageing, but rather a wide range of different ones, which, in combination, target successful ageing as a pluralistic and value-driven concept.

Health promotion and prevention policies are at the core of Rowe and Kahn's *pragmatic model* of successful ageing (Rowe & Kahn, 2015). The effectiveness of interventions improving the (functional) health of older people has been proven in empirical studies—for physical activity, for example (de Labra et al., 2015). If, however, health promotion measures rely on influencing individual behaviour to a similar magnitude across all members of the older population, inequalities in health will tend not to decrease, but will likely become even wider (Goldberg, 2012). Hence, health-related interventions driven by the pragmatic model must be well targeted in order to foster successful ageing not just for the affluent—who already enjoy the best odds of living long and healthy lives—but also for a wide range of diverse and disadvantaged societal groups.

According to the *hedonic model* of successful ageing, social policies should aim at improving life satisfaction and happiness in old age. As individual life satisfaction tends to remain strong until late in life (e.g. Gatz & Zarit, 1999; Wettstein et al., 2015; see, however, also the discussion in Kunzmann et al., 2000 and Schilling, 2006), it would seem a little difficult to improve substantially the subjective well-being of older citizenry via social policy. After all, differences in subjective well-being due to socio-economic status tend to be small (Pinquart & Sörensen, 2000). Although the notion of hedonic well-being might be an important one for social policy, it would not seem to represent an indicator sensitive enough help identify sections of the population in need of an improvement in their resource status. That said, one might expect that even small changes in the subjective well-being of a population could provide a signal to indicate substantial societal change. Hence, it may be worthwhile for policymakers to monitor subjective well-being over a wide variety of societal groups (Diener et al., 2009).

The criteria for successful ageing under *eudaimonic models* concern notions of personal growth and coping when faced with developmental challenges, using, for example, strategies of reminiscence (Pasupathi & Carstensen, 2003). Social policy could be used to support counselling and educational offerings so that older persons are equipped to deal with the developmental tasks of old age. Probably an even more important question is the ways in which the eudaimonic model might shape the values of decision-makers in the economy, society, and politics as their actions 'affect the well-being of those below them in the status hierarchies' (Ryff, 2018, p. 246). Hence, this model may serve as a driver for developing societal utopias, not only fulfilling economic objectives in areas like innovation and productivity, but also criteria based on encompassing indicators of well-being all through one's life course.

The general *capability model* was originally developed with a focus on social policy, initially with the aim of fighting poverty and improving opportunities to achieve a good quality of life in developing countries (Anand & Sen, 1997). Capability-based approaches are likely the only model that has found direct application in a wide range of social policy areas, for example in labour market policies (Bonvin, 2008), health policies (Stephens & Breheny, 2018), and in policies designed to promote inclusion for persons with disability (WHO, 2001). As capability-based approaches are inherently capable of incorporating both diversity in life goals and inequality in living situations, they can be used to help design policies for successful ageing, accounting for the heterogeneity that can be found in old age. One example of this might be policies aimed at promoting environments capable of assisting people to age successfully (see, for instance, policies on the creation of age-friendly cities, Beard & Petitot, 2010).

Policies driven by the *care ethics model* are not necessarily designed to pursue the ideal of successful ageing. In a sense, using the care ethics model in forming social policy would seem, at first glance, to provide merely a compensatory mechanism. However, the effort to maintain the autonomy and quality of life of the care recipient as a main objective of care policies can provide much more than simply state-driven compensation for loss of one's health and functioning. Rather than that, as we argued in Chapter 6, life phases that involve substantial care needs are currently on their way to becoming normative in nature, thus representing a 'life risk' that affects the many, rather than being restricted to a mere minority. In humanistic terms, providing support for this phase of life, and indeed actively designing how it is lived, seems an essential task, not least to maintain dignity in the final part of one's life cycle. By necessity, care providers—including not just relatives and nurses providing hands-on care, but also organizations arranging and supervising shelter and government agencies providing the funding and supervision of long-term care—play a central role in this context. Long-term care policies should be designed to help inspire change in the organization and practice of long-term care—from simply providing appropriate shelter to supporting the autonomy and quality of life of diverse groups of care recipients (Kane, 2001).

Examples for policies on successful ageing

There is as diverse a variety of social policies available to drive societal efforts to achieve successful ageing as there are definitions and models of successful ageing. The aim of such policies should be to combat social inequality and to enable a wide range of diverse groups of older people. Empirical evidence for the efficacy of social policies should rest on comparative research (e.g. Tesch-Römer & von Kondratowitz, 2006; Albert & Tesch-Römer, 2019). Evidence on policies in pursuit of successful ageing is scarce. Hence, we briefly present three (international) examples of policy initiatives that we see as being close to the aim of successful ageing, although they do not explicitly build on any of the models of successful ageing as elaborated in this book: policies for active ageing, polices for age-friendly cities, and policies for inclusive healthy ageing.

Policies for active ageing

The policy paradigm of 'active ageing' has been developed over the years in the European Union (Foster & Walker, 2015; Tesch-Römer, 2012; Tesch-Römer & Wurm, 2012). The European framework emphasizes the active participation of older persons in society, hence a policy aim that fits well with Rowe and Kahn's pragmatic definition of successful ageing. A major contribution in this context is the development of the Active Ageing Index (AAI), an instrument designed to provide data for use in comparative policy analysis (de São José et al., 2017; Zaidi et al., 2017). The index evaluates countries in relation to four domains (employment, volunteering, independent living, and enabling environments). In Europe, the Nordic countries are positioned in the upper third of the ranking, while the Central European countries and their Southern neighbours occupy places in the middle third, with the Eastern Europeans taking up the lower third of the ranking (Zaidi et al., 2017, p. 149). It has been shown that a country's gross domestic product per capita is positively related to its AAI score (r = .55; Zaidi et al., 2017, p. 152). As with all cross-sectional associations, however, the direction of the causal arrow is unclear—one cannot see whether greater societal wealth leads to better opportunities for active ageing or, vice versa, more active ageing leads to a more abundant societal wealth. Taking inequality into account, it could be shown that inequality in active ageing at the micro-level of the individual is negatively correlated with the average AAI at a macro-level (i.e. the country level). Countries with a low overall value for active ageing tend to have populations with greater inequalities in active ageing (Barslund et al., 2017). Hence, it may be that policies that invest in active ageing can do more than simply increase the overall participation of older adults in society: they may also help alleviate social inequality.

Policies for age-friendly cities

The policy approach centred on creating age-friendly cities puts greater emphasis on the spatial environment as a factor in successful ageing. The World Health Organization (WHO) defines the age-friendly city as one that adapts 'its structures and services to be accessible to and inclusive of older people with varying needs and capacities' (WHO, 2007, p. 1). Eight features provide the building blocks for an age-friendly city, three of which refer to a city's spatial environment and infrastructure: adequate outdoor spaces, public transportation, and housing, with the others being social participation, social inclusion, civic participation, and community support and health services. This description chimes well with the capability-based model of successful ageing, although it also has parallels with the care model in that optimal outdoor spaces and solutions for those with health impairments form part of its focus. Ideally, every age-friendly city should offer diverse opportunity structures to satisfy the needs of its diverse population of older people. At present, however, the enterprise of building age-friendly cities still looks more like a relatively intangible international movement than a firm and cohesive set of policies. This is largely owing to the vast diversity that can be seen in cities in both the developed and the developing world. Several factors for the success of creating an age-friendly city have been identified, including, for example, multi-stakeholder collaborations, government commitment, and the inclusion of older persons. However, there is, as yet, no conclusive evidence on precisely what elements contribute to such successes (Steels, 2015). Providing proper funding, however, seems to be a key problem in the effort to create age-friendly cities. After all, introducing subsidised public transport, building appropriate outdoor spaces, and improving housing all require substantial budgets (Fitzgerald & Caro, 2014). There is one decisive question whose answer will determine whether an age-friendly city fulfils the expectations set for it: does it enable all older people—rich and poor—to live their lives according to the individual values and wishes each of them aspires to pursue. Empirical evidence on the outcomes of efforts to create age-friendly cities is rather scarce, however, although some studies in the area of community gerontology have revealed some of the influential factors in the environment that affect successful ageing (Greenfield et al., 2019).

Policies for healthy ageing

The WHO recently declared a Decade of Healthy Ageing, which is to last from 2020 to 2030 (WHO, 2020a). The definition of 'healthy ageing' that forms the focus of this decade of activity is given as 'the process of developing and maintaining the functional ability that enables well-being in older age' (WHO, 2020b, p. 8). By this definition, the absence of disease or infirmity is not a requirement for healthy ageing, as many older adults will suffer from one or more health conditions that, if controlled appropriately, will have little influence on their well-being. Thus, this approach is in accordance with both the capability-based and the care ethics approach to successful ageing, with an emphasis on integrating as diverse as possible a range of ageing trajectories. Since the international Decade of Healthy Ageing has only just begun, it is too early to expect any concrete results from it. Nevertheless, it can already be said that any strategies for improvement will be built on the basis of a combination of insights gleaned from examples of best practice together with more rigorous comparative research on the effects of national policies on healthy ageing (WHO, 2020b).

Granting access to successful ageing by tackling life-long inequality

Social inequality poses one of the most fundamental challenges to the objective of achieving successful ageing for each and every older person. As we have seen time and again, access to valuable resources has a close connection with leading a healthy, happy, and fulfilled life. Hence, welfare state policies should consist not only in interventions for successful ageing in general, but also take into consideration the diverse needs of those who have no access to high-value resources. In addition, policies for successful ageing need to embrace the diversity within ageing, not only with respect to gender, as shown in this chapter, but also to race (Ferraro et al., 2017) and sexual orientation (Fabbre, 2015). Finally, ageing societies need to achieve a culture change: in order to create opportunity for successful ageing, we need to change the way we think, feel, and act towards age and ageing (WHO, 2020b). And precisely this challenge is the topic of the next chapter.

PART III

AMBIVALENCES
AND AMBITIONS
OF SUCCESSFUL AGEING

8

Successful ageing and ageism

A bidirectional model of influence

Liat Ayalon

In contrast to the common negative stereotypes that represent ageing and old age as a period of inevitable decline, disease, and deteriorating functioning, the concept of successful ageing offers a more positive outlook, with nuances of longevity and eternal youth (see Chapter 1). Nevertheless, regardless of the exact model of successful ageing that one has in focus, the notion itself is fundamentally ageist in that it promotes a normative dichotomy between successful and unsuccessful older people by explicitly implying that some older adults age successfully, while others fail to meet a desirable standard in the way in which they grow old. To date, much of the criticism of the concept has been pointed at the Rowe and Kahn (1997) model, which is thought to place responsibility for successful ageing in the hands of the individual, largely disregarding societal influences on one's ageing process (Calasanti, 2016). As we discuss in this chapter, even the wider notion of successful ageing itself merits some criticism on the basis of the meanings implied by the term. This chapter begins by describing the ageist features inherent in Rowe and Kahn's successful ageing model, but then moves on to describe ageism as a barrier to successful ageing, regardless of a specific model for success one has in focus. It concludes by listing some recommendations on how best to refine the concept and on possible changes in policy.

Why is the concept successful ageing ageist?

Ageism is defined as the harbouring of stereotypes and prejudice against people and discriminating against them as a result of their age. Ageism can have both a positive and a negative side, and can be directed towards people of any age group. Ageism can be directed towards others (other-directed ageism) and/or towards oneself (self-directed ageism), and can be expressed either explicitly or implicitly, with limited or no awareness of being ageist in one's speech or behaviour (Ayalon & Tesch-Römer, 2018a). Ageism hurts older people because it prevents them from reaching their full potential, both by explicitly determining what older people can and cannot do, and by implicitly impacting on older people's perceptions of their own ageing process (Ayalon & Tesch-Römer, 2018a). Ageism may also interact with sexism and racism, thus exacerbating disadvantages, especially in older age (Collins et al., 2017).

The term 'successful ageing' bluntly divides the ageing population into successes and failures (McLaughlin et al., 2010). This binary categorization tends to regard most older adults as having failed to age successfully. Past research has found that 21.1 per cent of Danish citizens over the age of 65 years, but only 1.6 per cent of Polish people, can be classified as successful agers, based on Rowe and Kahn's definition (Hank, 2011). It would seem clear, then, that the classification poses unattainable standards for the majority of older adults (Tesch-Römer & Wahl, 2017). Ignoring the diversity of older people and disregarding the fact that, although average lifespans have increased, compression of comorbidity has been slower to occur, a failure that poses a number of problems and that may serve as an instigator of ageism (Jönson, 2013). This work argues that the notion of successful ageing poses the danger of replacing extremely negative biomedical stereotypes of ageing and old age with extremely positive ones, many of which turn out to be unrealistic and out of reach of the majority of older people.

Whereas early depictions of older adults in the media have been largely negative, emphasizing suffering and disability, that portrayal has since shifted to represent far more positive, successful models of ageing, representing an over-idealistic vision of old age (Loos & Ivan, 2018). In the effort to portray a message of successful ageing, older adults are often presented as if they were extremely fit, healthy, and happy middle-agers (Gewirtz-Meydan & Ayalon, 2018). This representation belies the great variability of older people (Loos & Ivan, 2018). Moreover, such imagery will tend to prevent older people from accepting and acknowledging the decline that may well be an inevitable part of the ageing process.

The distinction between the Third Age, which closely resembles middle age—and is thus used to characterize 'successful ageing'—and the Fourth Age, which is characterized by decline and disability—and thus represents 'failure'—ends up producing both other- and self-directed ageism (Higgs & Gilleard, 2020). To be more specific, studies have shown that older adults often do not see themselves as old (Minichiello et al., 2000) and do not identify with their peers owing to the negative social status allocated to old age (Chonody & Teater, 2016). This can result in social isolation and loneliness among older adults (Ayalon, 2018). Moreover, past research has attributed some of the reluctance of some older adults to use long-term care services to an ageist attitude towards other older adults (Dobbs et al., 2008).

This exact same negative approach taken towards others seen as having failed to comply with the established model of successful ageing can also be turned against oneself. In a society that emphasizes successful models of ageing, failing to meet the ideal can be looked upon as a personal failure (Calasanti et al., 2018). The entire beauty industry is built around such a concept as it actively advocates for one to make a conscious effort toward off signs of ageing and ensure that one continues to look and feel as young as possible for as long as possible (Katz, 2001). Failing to meet such unattainable standards, in addition to leaving one socially invisible (Clarke & Griffin, 2008) can give rise to feelings of dissatisfaction, contempt, and resentment towards oneself. This has shown to have deleterious effects, particularly on women (Clarke & Griffin, 2008).

Just as Rowe and Kahn's model of successful ageing model implied that the outcomes of one's process of ageing is in one's own hands, it might be said that any falling short of the unattainable standards set for one is a personal failure (Calasanti, 2016; Calasanti & King, 2020). If society assigns volition and agency to one's functional and cognitive states, then it is easy for it to disregard the role of cumulative advantages and disadvantages in people's lives (Calasanti, 2016; Calasanti & King, 2020). Past research has shown a dramatic variability in the ways in which people age. For instance, a consistent education-related gradient can be seen from the research, suggesting that those among us who enjoy higher levels of education also enjoy better health and a longer lifespan (Präg et al., 2017). Similar gradients have been observed in relation to race and ethnicity, and in relation to childhood socio-economic status (Cohen et al., 2010; Robert & Ruel, 2006). The choice of a neo-liberal attitude—one that views old age as the product of one's own initiative and efforts—allows one to disregard societal influences. Such a stance can be quite depreciatory towards those among us who have failed to meet the desired outcome for successful ageing.

Why does ageism prevent people from ageing successfully?

Although the term 'successful ageing' is problematic, and some models and visions of successful ageing are deserving of criticism, the term does have the virtue that it encompasses a variety of desired ageing experiences and outcomes. These may include not only the aim of living a longer and healthier life, but also of being surrounded by one's family and friends, living a meaningful life, or being content and satisfied with one's life. All these various characteristics that can be grouped under the generic term 'successful ageing' are prone to being impacted upon by the harmful effects of ageism on the lives of older people (Ayalon & Tesch-Römer, 2018b). Hence, it is important to note not only that the Rowe and Kahn model of successful ageing, or even the notion of 'successful ageing' itself, can encourage ageism as a by-product, but may also even pose a barrier to ageing successfully or to ageing in some other desirable way.

Past research has identified three pathways by which ageism can hamper one's ability to age successfully (Swift et al., 2017). The first is through age-based discrimination, which can impact negatively on people's health and well-being. To be more specific, age-based discrimination may result in poorer services being allocated to older people simply by virtue of their age. In turn, this can result in poorer health for those who are victims of this type of discrimination (Levy et al., 2020). Age-based discrimination may also impact people's well-being as it is interpreted as a negative event maliciously directed towards a person due to his or her age (Lyons et al., 2018). Of note is the fact that age-based discrimination may intersect with other characteristics such as gender, race, and physical ability, and thus differentially impacting on the ageing process of different population groups (Krekula et al., 2018; McGann et al., 2016).

A second pathway that may pose a barrier to people ageing successfully is that of one's own self-perceptions of the process of ageing. Young children acquire certain beliefs about and stereotypes towards ageing and old age very early in their lives. As people grow old, these stereotypes, which those people have internalized throughout their lives, can begin to act as self-fulfilling prophecies (Levy, 2009). Individuals who hold more negative views about their own ageing process are more likely to age poorly and be less likely to engage in self-care activities and healthy behaviours (Levy & Myers, 2004). They are also more prone to falls (Ayalon, 2016), to medical comorbidity and depression, and are more likely even to die earlier than peers who hold more positive views of their ageing process (Kotter-Grühn et al., 2009). Hence, self-ageism (i.e. ageism directed towards oneself), as manifested in negative self-perceptions of ageing, may hamper one's ability to age successfully.

The stereotype threat, an expression that refers to concerns about the consequences of conforming to negative stereotypes of one's own social group, represents another pathway through which a person's efforts to age successfully might be hampered (Swift et al., 2017). Whereas stereotype embodiment theory accounts for the internalization of age-related stereotypes throughout one's lifespan and the ways in which old-age stereotypes become relevant to oneself as one ages, the stereotype threat model suggests that merely finding oneself in situations that trigger age-related stereotypes can increase one's likelihood of conforming to such stereotypes as a result of increased strain and anxiety. For instance, once a person is in a situation that activates age stereotypes, they may become increasingly anxious and thus begin to conform to stereotypes simply because the situation increased their sense of threat. Research has shown that older people tend to underperform in certain cognitive tasks under conditions of stereotype threat, thus confirming negative stereotypes related to the decline in cognitive functioning in old age (Barber & Mather, 2013).

Implications for concept refinement and policy

The notion of 'successful ageing' has generated a change in societal discourse and thinking. It has opened the door to a new approach towards seeing old age and older people as capable and thriving. However, we think it is time to elaborate yet further on perceptions of old age by including the entire spectrum of ageing experiences in our analysis (Tesch-Römer & Wahl, 2017). Adopting an inclusive approach is likely to result in reduced ageism as it is likely to highlight the variability in the experience of old age. Such an approach will help facilitate people to identify with and accept a variety of trajectories of ageing and old age, and thereby reduce the level of ageism directed both against oneself and against others.

There have been many calls over the years for a change in the terminology used to describe, and the meaning ascribed to the concept of, successful ageing in order to make the concept more inclusive towards people from a wide variety of sociocultural backgrounds (Liang & Luo, 2012) and a broad range of physical and cognitive abilities. The underlying desire is to inspire an inclusive model that avoids dichotomizing individuals as belonging to either the 'success' or the 'failure' category. Any such approach should be process-rather than outcome-oriented in order to ensure that the needs of older adults are satisfied, while respecting their autonomy and dignity, no matter what their age and/or level of ability may be (Tesch-Römer & Wahl, 2017).

It seems essential to move from a neo-liberal approach to a model that acknowledges the role of the environment and society in people's ageing experiences (Calasanti & King, 2020). Such an approach may be expected to acknowledge that cumulative advantages and disadvantages throughout our lives are important factors in preventing or promoting positive or negative experiences in ageing. An emphasis needs to be placed on intersectionality to provide a better understanding of how age interacts with other social statuses, including gender, education, and wealth, throughout one's lifespan (Warner & Brown, 2011).

Finally, some emphasis needs to be placed on the significant toll that ageism takes on people's quality of life and its impact on the ageing experience (Levy et al., 2020). To be in a position to live in a society well suited to all ages, it is essential that we change the way we think, feel, and act towards people by virtue of their age (Ayalon, 2020). Past research has shown that imparting knowledge about ageism, educating people on the phenomenon, and fostering contact between the generations can be effective in reducing ageist attitudes (Burnes et al., 2019). We also know that explicit laws and regulations banning discrimination based on age can help change societal norms and behaviours (Neumark et al., 2019). Hence, although the concept of successful ageing needs some refinement before it can be capable of acknowledging the full variety of ageing trajectories, it is important to ensure that older people live in a world in which they have the chance to realize their full potential and in which they are considered an integral part of society.

9

Towards a new narrative
on successful ageing

So, are there any promising pathways open to us to arrive at some sort of reconciliation between the very divergent positions and perspectives on successful ageing that we have outlined in this book? Our answer to this question, at least as we describe it in this closing chapter, is threefold in that (1) we emphasize the need for pluralism in conceptual reasoning on the notion of successful ageing; (2) we insist that one must be aware of the full implications of choosing any particular model of successful ageing; and (3) we assert that the discourse on successful ageing can only, to a limited extent, be driven by empirical data, but must also be illuminated by an understanding of the underlying normative conceptions of what it means to enjoy a good life in old age. In this closing chapter of our book, taking its title at face value, although reversing the order of the notions listed in its subtitle, we begin by discussing the ambivalences in the term and then go on to tackle its ambitions. But, first of all, we bring together a list of what we consider to be the most fundamental questions related to the concept of successful ageing (in Box 9.1).

Ambivalences of the concept of successful ageing

The concept of successful ageing can clearly, as we have outlined in several of the previous chapters, produces mixed feelings, both hope and dread, both excitement and anger. In the next few paragraphs, we summarize what we see as the main positive and negative points of the concept, either as inherent features of the notion of successful ageing or as potential implications of its use.

Successful ageing promises to be a unifying term, but it has countless definitions

A first ambivalence that we detect is located in the exaggerated optimism that one has finally come to terms with the many definitions of successful ageing.

Box 9.1. Successful ageing: ambivalences and ambitions

Ambivalences in the concept of successful ageing
- Successful ageing promises to be a unifying term, but it has countless definitions.
- Successful ageing provides indicators that turn out to be rather fuzzy markers of ageing well.
- Successful ageing directs attention to heterogeneity in old age but oversimplifies that heterogeneity.
- Successful ageing gives hope but may also have the effect of increasing ageism.

Ambitions of the concept of successful ageing
- Successful ageing provides a vision for what it is to lead a good life in old age.
- Successful ageing models help bring to the surface values related to ageing well.
- Successful ageing infuses life-course views of ageing.
- Successful ageing fosters a contextual view of the process of getting older.
- Successful ageing helps one to remain aware of social inequalities.
- Successful ageing can help inform social policies on life courses and ageing.

In their seminal review of the literature, Depp and Jeste (2006) arrived at 29 definitions based on 28 studies. Yet from the literature available 7 years later, Cosco et al. (2013) extracted as many as 105 operational definitions, based on 84 studies. The quest to find a robust and generally accepted definition in accord with the standards of best practice in (ageing) science, one that contains and preserves the best of the concept and leaves behind all the controversial parts of the notion, now seems to be the ultimate goal in the current discourse on successful ageing. Certainly, one has to applaud the requirement that Pruchno (2015) insisted to use the concept of successful ageing in a straightforward manner within ageing science. Pruchno wrote that 'it is incumbent on gerontologists to use the conceptual and empirical knowledge base that now exists to develop consensus about what successful ageing is and how it should be measured' (2015, p. 3). Although we are inclined to agree with Pruchno's claim, we doubt the consensus it demands would be a realistic goal to hope for, a doubt that is reinforced by the multiplicity of conflicting values behind the many models of successful ageing that we have described throughout this book.

Successful ageing provides indicators that turn out to be rather fuzzy markers of ageing well

It is an uncomfortable real-world fact that rates of successful ageing traced empirically in studies employing differing conceptualizations of successful ageing can vary from as little as 0.04 per cent to as much as 95 per cent (Depp

& Jeste, 2006). Even looking at self-evaluations, the number of older adults who see their own ageing path as being successful have varied in available studies between 50 per cent and 92 per cent (Timonen, 2016). Both of these hugely deviating ranges in results are clearly unsatisfactory for any scientific concept expected to yield validly and reliably measured metrics. Imagine a definition for depression that rationally leads to a number of different assessment instruments, some of which identify practically nobody as being depressed and others that characterize almost everybody as suffering from the illness. It would not take long for such a concept to be discarded. So, what to do? As we see it, while empirical data are important, successful ageing is an area in which data absolutely *must* be framed against particular models of successful ageing. It could be argued that there is always a need to undertake such a conceptual framing in empirical ageing science, but in the arena of successful ageing, with its direct implications on what it means to enjoy a good life in old age, the exercise of framing the data conceptually, and of placing it in relation to the values upon which such frames are based, becomes utterly essential. Data on rates of depression may not always demand that the reader be told precisely what underlying notion of depression is being employed because there is fairly broad consensus on what depression actually is. This is simply not the case in successful ageing and just quoting rates of successful ageing given in publications or public discussions will inevitably be misleading unless one explicitly outlines the theory and value orientations underlying such figures. Where empirical discrepancies emerge, it becomes necessary to build theoretical linkages between the differing worldviews on what it means to age successfully. Hence, scientists who make use of the concept of successful ageing should be aware of these issues and in presenting their results should make transparent their theoretical choices on the underlying definition of successful ageing, both to fellow scientists and to political audiences and the general public.

Successful ageing directs attention to heterogeneity in old age but oversimplifies that heterogeneity

Heterogeneity—i.e. differences between individuals—increases with age at many levels. The increase can, for example, be seen in areas such as in cognitive functioning, social relations, multiple morbidity, and activities of daily life (Maddox, 1987; Mitnitski et al., 2017; Nelson & Dannefer, 1992). The pronounced heterogeneity in ageing processes and outcomes may be due to increasing social inequality (Ferraro & Shippee, 2009), to increasing diversity in lifestyles and in life course trajectories (Daatland & Biggs, 2006), to the accumulation of biographical experiences specific to each individual, or to biological changes at various levels, from genetics to organ functioning. We argue that the discourse on successful ageing may have the effect of hindering understanding of this heterogeneity in ageing for two primary reasons: Firstly, the concept of successful ageing reinforces a dualistic discourse in ageing research. The distinction made by Neugarten (1974) between the young-old and old-old, for example, has had major scientific reverberations and yet has stigmatized large groups of older adults ever since (Ehni & Wahl, 2020). We fear that the same is likely to be true of the notion of successful ageing. Secondly, we also fear that using the concept of successful ageing leaves us open to the danger of narrowing 'ageing lifestyles' down merely to the accepted and socially approved norms of what it is to enjoy a good life in old age. Support for such a norm runs the risk of neglecting the heterogeneity of old age and of dulling down the rich colour to be found in the differing pathways of ageing by the accepting narrow and one-sided expectations of successful ageing among individuals and societies in the future.

Successful ageing not only gives hope, but may also have the effect of increasing ageism

Seeing successful ageing as the only desirable norm for the ageing process will have the effect of devaluing life courses that do not comply with that norm and can hence lead to an attitude that increases ageism (see also Chapter 8). Although ageism may be both positive and negative, its negative side appears much more frequently. Any decision to employ the concept of successful ageing can end up having contradictory effects in the long run: propagating successful ageing as the norm may undermine already low rates of successful ageing by broadening the range of pathways along which the adverse outcomes of ageism and age discrimination can unfold. Hence, any such direction would require performing a difficult balancing act between avoiding the trap of ageism and realizing the potentials of successful ageing.

Ambitions of the concept of successful ageing

Although we can clearly see the ambivalences associated with the concept of successful ageing, we believe that the ambitions of the concepts are attractive enough to justify retaining the term as one of the key concepts of ageing research. However, according to our argument, doing so can only yield useful results if we restrict ourselves rigorously to what the concept is capable of offering—and to avoid interpretations that are heuristically unfruitful, misleading, overstretching the case, or merely wishful thinking. We go on now to sketch the ambitions of the concept.

Successful ageing provides a vision for what it is to lead a good life in old age

Following many scholars in the field of successful ageing (e.g., Pruchno, 2015; Rowe & Kahn, 1997, 2015), we argue that the task of counteracting the deficit model of ageing remains a formidable challenge both to gerontology and to wider society in an ageing world. We need visions of what it means to enjoy a good life in old age. One example of such a vision is the World Health Organization's (WHO) concept of healthy ageing. As already mentioned, the WHO has declared the decade 2020–2030 as the Decade of Healthy Ageing (WHO, 2020b). We recommend seeing the conceptualization of healthy ageing not as being in competition with the concept of successful ageing, but instead as recognizing the large amount of productive overlap between the two notions. Put briefly, the concept of healthy ageing contains all the important elements of models of successful ageing, although its focus is on 'health in life'. In contrast, successful ageing has a strong connection with health, with its focus being on 'life in health'. Thus, the two concepts together seem to provide a complementary vision of the good life in old age.

Successful ageing models help bring to the surface values related to ageing well

There can be no discourse on successful ageing without establishing a discourse on the values according to which one may judge what it means to enjoy a good life. We propose that use of the term 'successful ageing' in conceptual, as well as empirical, studies should always be looked upon as an essential part of discussions on (in places conflicting) values in models of successful ageing (Ryff, 2018). That said, we hope our value-driven classification of models of successful ageing will be of help to researchers, practitioners, political actors, and ageing laypeople alike to become more keenly aware of the value implications of favouring one model of successful ageing over another (see Chapter 3). Hence, the challenge is to make value-informed decisions and thereby come to terms with the value choices needed in these post-modern times about what it is to enjoy a good life in old age. However, acknowledging the need for value-informed decision-making on models goes together with an acceptance of pluralism about the available concepts of successful ageing and therefore with accepting a generous level of multi-finality in how one may achieve successful ageing. As researchers, practitioners, and political actors, we have at our disposal a diverse range of conceptions on successful ageing to choose from, anchored in equally diverse—and sometimes contradictory—value systems. The fact that we have established such diversity in ageing may be seen as among the greatest achievements of modern societies experiencing a number of far-reaching demographic transitions. We would therefore regard any attempt to use the concept of successful ageing as a means of narrowing such diversity back down again as both counterproductive and politically retrogressive. However, this does not mean that either an 'anything goes' or a 'just let it go' conclusion would necessarily be the consequence. On the contrary: we are required to make choices, and we need to be aware of the implications and consequences of choosing one model over another.

Successful ageing infuses life-course views of ageing

Ageing is part of one's life course. Hence, all the models of successful ageing that we have discussed in this book (see Chapter 3) need to be looked at from a life-course perspective. We need to collect more empirical evidence on how long- and short-term connections unfold over the full course of one's life. Yet the fascinating research already in existence that looks at the long-term consequences of prenatal and early childhood experiences has not yet been linked very strongly with empirical research on successful ageing. Aside from that, Mathilda Riley's argument that the flow of the typical life course is likely to undergo dramatic changes in the future carries with it enormous consequences for the debate on successful ageing (Riley & Riley, 2000). Riley argued that the classic flow of events from education to work and then to leisure is soon quite likely to no longer suit the needs of postmodern societies. We strongly believe that future debates on successful ageing are closely linked to debates on changes to the ways in which life courses are institutionalized and in which traditional life-course patterns are likely to be deinstitutionalized (Settersten, 2017). At a psychological and biological level, longitudinal data covering very long observational periods are now available to support the idea that successful ageing begins in childhood and early life, and that it is already being shaped long before a person is even close to being 'old'. Biological ageing is a hugely diverse phenomenon, as is the extent of biological ageing early in life, together with signs of early dementia, stroke, and of other more 'unsuccessful' personal futures in general (Belsky et al., 2015). It has also been shown that differences between individuals as early as at the age of 11 years can predict cognitive functioning, health outcomes, and even mortality at the age of 80 (Deary et al., 2004). A range of adversities in early life has a negative association with measurements of well-being in old age (Schafer et al., 2011). To summarize, the data accumulating on the 'long arm' of early biopsychosocial risk factors for late successful ageing are already quite impressive (see also Wahl, 2016).

Successful ageing fosters a contextual view of the process of getting older

The contexts in which older people live—contexts provided by homes, neighbourhoods, and municipalities, as well as by modern technology—have been spelled out repeatedly in our arguments here. That emphasis brings with it a series of benefits for our understanding of the concept of successful ageing and its impact both on individuals and on societies. Firstly, it counteracts the dominant tendency in the existing literature to conceptualize successful ageing as being largely a phenomenon of the individual, a view that seems to be becoming increasingly outdated in light of the empirical data on the contexts of ageing accumulated over the last 20 years or so (Wahl & Gerstorf, 2018). Secondly, the emphatic inclusion of care contexts into the equation opens out new ways of defining successful ageing even in situations of severe frailty that so typically arise in advanced old age. This does not force one to accept that successful ageing can only be understood as completely arbitrary, but it might just lead one to consider adding a range of new criteria for different conceptions of successful ageing. It is evident that more intervention-oriented research is needed to underpin this educated hunch with empirical data, as we are currently not at all sure of the extent to which further improved care contexts, optimized assistive technology, and adaptive home environments have the capacity to bring benefits to people with major care needs in the future. Research work based on a care-oriented model of successful ageing has the potential to be particularly relevant, not just to older people and family caregivers, but also to professional nurses, geriatric professionals, and policymakers.

Successful ageing helps one to remain aware of social inequalities

There has been considerable criticism in the past, and indeed at the present time, of the fact that the concept of successful ageing is clearly affected by a range of social inequalities and that it has an unfortunate tendency to foster the viewpoints of ageing elites (Calasanti & King, 2020; Hank, 2011). The task of defining the standards of what constitutes a good life in old age—a major ambition of discourses on successful ageing—may also be seen as a way of pointing to existing social inequalities as sharply as possible, in matters of health and health care, and in life expectancy, for example. In other words, highlighting models of successful ageing that spell out the values governing what one should aim to achieve as one's developmental goal or, as some would put it, what counts as 'successful development' (Haase et al., 2013), will likely have the effect of highlighting even further the role of social inequality in ageing well.

Successful ageing can help inform social policies on the life courses and ageing

The discourse on successful ageing can play a major role in achieving a better understanding of the interconnections within life at its micro-, meso-, and macro-layers. For instance, one's community provides a resource-rich meso-level that can be particularly helpful in forming connections from the micro- to the macro-level (Greenfield et al., 2019). At the macro-level of politics, opportunity structures for social engagement, to adopt Rowe and Kahn's (1997) term, can impact quite directly on individuals. And remaining on the macro-level of whole societies, models of successful ageing can provide important tools for formulating policies to intervene in people's life courses and to help people to age well. Social policies have the potential to foster good health, active participation, and even happiness among older people. Not only would this allow individual ageing trajectories to be shaped positively, but it may also help societies in their pursuit of a 'demographic dividend' (Olshansky et al., 2007).

Conclusion

We conclude our book by revealing the choice for the meme on the cover of the book, a mythological depiction of a being with three faces. This sculpture embellishes the 'Temple of Friendship' in the palace garden of Schloss Schönbusch in Bavaria. Looking in three different directions, we would like to leave our readers with three questions and three tentative answers, showing that an effort to push the discourse on successful ageing forward may turn out to be fruitful both in conducting future ageing research and in intervening on the practical conditions that impact upon ageing well.

Our first question addresses how one might best use the concept of successful ageing going forward. Should we abandon the concept of successful ageing altogether or take best advantage of it in academia and societal discourse in future? We hope to have by now convincingly shown that the term successful ageing will remain one of the core constructs of ageing research. Nevertheless, we remain very aware of the ambivalences that emanate from it, and hence of the need to take great care in our use of it.

Our second question relates to the need for an acceptable definition of successful ageing with the potential to unify. Is there a need for us to decide on some particular model of successful ageing once and for all? The conclusion we have come to is that the diversity and heterogeneity of old age renders it essential to look at successful ageing from a pluralistic perspective and hence to use the full variety of models of successful ageing as a portfolio of values to govern what constitutes enjoying a good life in old age.

Our third and final question relates to the ambitions and ambivalences associated with the various concepts of successful ageing. Is the immediate and visionary potential of the concept of successful ageing stronger than the risk it poses of doing harm to the process of ageing and to older people? To be honest, we have no definitive answer to this question based on what we discussed in this book. Any concept of successful ageing is forced to rely on normative judgements that value some pathways into old age and devalue others. Any call to shape these judgements toward a uniform direction in order to foster the notion of successful ageing may be (too) high a price to pay. Still, the ambition of ageing successfully—to remain healthy and happy, to develop one's wisdom, and to be and feel well supported and cared for—should be seen as helpful for creating developmental opportunities and avoiding developmental risks into old and very old age.

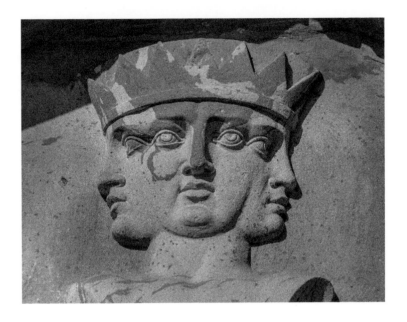

References

Albert, I., & Tesch-Römer, C. (2019). Cross-cultural psychogerontology. In S. Wurm & A. E. Kornadt (Eds.), Encyclopedia of gerontology and population aging (pp. 1–6). Springer. https://doi.org/10.1007/978-3-319-69892-2_95-1

Anand, S., & Sen, A. (1997). Concepts of human development and poverty: a multidimensional perspective. In United Nations Development Programme (Ed.), Poverty and human development: human development papers 1997 (pp. 1–20). UNDP.

Antonucci, T. C., Fiori, K. L., Birditt, K. S., & Jackey, L. M. H. (2010). Convoys of social relations: integrating life-span and life-course perspectives. In R. M. Lerner, M. E. Lamb, & A. M. Freund (Eds), The handbook of life-span development (Vol. 2, pp. 434–473). Wiley. https://doi.org/doi: 10.1002/9780470880166.hlsd002012

Antonucci, T. C., Birditt, K. S., & Ajrouch, K. (2011). Convoys of s+ocial relations: past, present, and future. In K. L. Fingerman, C. A. Berg, J. Smith, & T. C. Antonucci (Eds), Handbook of life-span development (pp. 161–182). Springer Publishing.

Antonucci, T. C., Ajrouch, K. J., & Birditt, K. S. (2014). The convoy model: explaining social relations from a multidisciplinary perspective. The Gerontologist, 54(1), 82–92. https://doi.org/doi:10.1093/geront/gnt118

Assmann, J. (2005). Das kulturelle Gedächtnis: Schrift, Erinnerung und politische Identität in frühen Hochkulturen [Cultural heritage: scripture, remembering and political identity] (5th ed.). Beck.

Ausserhofer, D., Deschodt, M., De Geest, S., van Achterberg, T., Meyer, G., Verbeek, H., Sjetne, I. S., Malinowska-Lipień, I., Griffiths, P., Schlüter, W., & Engberg, S. (2016). 'There's no place like home': a scoping review on the impact of homelike residential care models on resident-, family-, and staff-related outcomes. Journal of the American Medical Directors Association, 17, 685–693. https://doi.org/doi:10.1016/j.jamda.2016.03.009

Ayalon, L. (2016). Satisfaction with aging results in reduced risk for falling. International Psychogeriatrics, 28, 741–747. https://doi.org/10.1017/S1041610215001969

Ayalon, L. (2018). Loneliness and anxiety about aging in adult day care centers and continuing care retirement communities. Innovation in Aging, 2, igy021. https://doi.org/https://doi.org/ https://doi.org/10.1093/geroni/igy021

Ayalon, L. (2020). Life in a world for all ages: from a utopic idea to reality. Journal of Elder Policy, 1, 39–67. https://doi.org/doi:10.18278/jep.1.1.3

Ayalon, L., & Tesch-Römer, C. (Eds). (2018a). Contemporary perspectives on ageism. Springer. https://doi.org/doi: 10.1007/978-3-319-73820-8.

Ayalon, L., & Tesch-Römer, C. (2018b). Ageism: concept and origins. In L. Ayalon & C. Tesch-Römer (Eds), Contemporary perspectives on ageism (pp. 1–10). Springer.

Baird, B. M., Lucas, R. E., & Donnellan, M. B. (2010). Life satisfaction across the life-span: findings from two nationally representative panel studies. *Social Indicators Research*, 99, 183–203. https://doi.org/10.1007/s11205-010-9584-9

Baltes, P. B., & Baltes, M. M. (1990a). *Successful aging: perspectives from the behavioral sciences*. Cambridge University Press. https://doi.org/10.1017/CBO9780511665684

Baltes, P. B., & Baltes, M. M. (1990b). Psychological perspectives on successful aging: the model of selective optimization with compensation. In P. B. Baltes & M. M. Baltes (Eds), *Successful aging: perspectives from the behavioral sciences* (pp. 1–34). Cambridge University Press. https://doi.org/10.1017/CBO9780511665684.003

Baltes, P. B., & Staudinger, U. M. (2000). Wisdom: a metaheuristic (pragmatic) to orchestrate mind and virtue toward excellence. *American Psychologist*, 55, 122–136. https://doi.org/10.1037/0003-066X.55.1.122

Baltes, P. B., & Smith, J. (2003). New frontiers in the future of aging: from successful aging of the young old to the dilemmas of the fourth age. *Gerontology*, 49, 123–135. https://doi.org/10.1159/000067946

Baltes, M. M., Wahl, H.-W., & Reichert, M. (1991). Successful aging in long-term care institutions. *Annual Review of Gerontology and Geriatrics*, 11, 311–337.

Baltes, P. B., Lindenberger, U., & Staudinger, U. M. (2006). Life span theory in developmental psychology. In W. Damon & R. M. Lerner (Eds), *Handbook of child psychology: volume 1. Theoretical models of human development* (pp. 569–664). Wiley. https://doi.org/10.1002/9780470147658.chpsy0111

Banks, J., Marmot, M., Oldfield, Z., & Smith, J. P. (2009). The SES health gradient on both sides of the atlantic. In D. A. Wise (Ed.), *Developments in the economics of aging* (pp. 359–406). University of Chicago Press https://doi.org/http://www.nber.org/chapters/c11324

Barber, S. J., & Mather, M. (2013). Stereotype threat can both enhance and impair older adults' memory. *Psychological Science*, 24, 2522–2529. https://doi.org/10.1177/0956797613497023

Barslund, M., Von Werder, M., & Zaidi, A. (2017). Inequality in active ageing: evidence from a new individual-level index for European countries. *Ageing & Society*, 39, 541–567. https://doi.org/10.1017/S0144686X17001052

Bauman, A., Merom, D., Bull, F. C., Buchner, D. M., & Fiatarone Singh, M. A. (2016). Updating the evidence for physical activity: summative reviews of the epidemiological evidence, prevalence, and interventions to promote 'active aging'. *The Gerontologist*, 56(Suppl._2), S268–S280. https://doi.org/10.1093/geront/gnw031

Baumeister, R. F., & Leary, M. R. (1995). The need to belong: desire for interpersonal attachments as a fundamental human motivation. *Psychological Bulletin*, 117, 497–529. https://doi.org/10.1037/0033-2909.117.3.497

Beard, J. R., & Petitot, C. (2010). Ageing and urbanization: can cities be designed to foster active ageing? *Public Health Reviews*, 32, 427–450. https://doi.org/10.1007/BF03391610

Belsky, D. W., Caspi, A., Houts, R., Cohen, H. J., Corcoran, D. L., Danese, A., Harrington, H., Israel, S., Levine, M. E., & Schaefer, J. D. (2015). Quantification of biological aging in young adults. *Proceedings of the National Academy of*

Sciences, 112, E4104–E4110. https://doi.org/www.pnas.org/cgi/doi/10.1073/pnas.1506264112

Beltrán-Sánchez, H., Razak, F., & Subramanian, S. V. (2014). Going beyond the disability-based morbidity definition in the compression of morbidity framework. *Global Health Action, 7,* 24766. https://doi.org/10.3402/gha.v7.24766

Biernat, E., & Piatkowska, M. (2018). Stay active for life: physical activity across life stages. *Clinical Interventions in Aging, 13,* 1341–1352. https://doi.org/10.2147/CIA.S167131

Binstock, R. H. (2003). The war on 'anti-aging medicine'. *The Gerontologist, 43,* 4–14. https://doi.org/10.1093/geront/43.1.4

Bonvin, J.-M. (2008). Activation policies, new modes of governance and the issue of responsibility. *Social Policy and Society, 7*(3), 367–377. https://doi.org/10.1017/S1474746408004338

Bosnes, I., Nordahl, H. M., Stordal, E., Bosnes, O., Myklebust, T. Å., & Almkvist, O. (2019). Lifestyle predictors of successful aging: a 20-year prospective HUNT study. *PLoS ONE, 14,* e0219200. https://doi.org/10.1371/journal.pone.0219200

Brandt, M., Deindl, C., & Hank, K. (2012). Tracing the origins of successful aging: the role of childhood conditions and social inequality in explaining later life health. *Social Science and Medicine, 74,* 1418–1425. https://doi.org/10.1016/j.socscimed.2012.01.004

Brandtstädter, J. (2009). Goal pursuit and goal adjustment: self-regulation and intentional self-development in changing developmental contexts. *Advances in Life Course Research, 14,* 52–62. https://doi.org/10.1016/j.alcr.2009.03.002

Brandtstädter, J., & Renner, G. (1990). Tenacious goal pursuit and flexible goal adjustment: explication and age-related analysis of assimilative and accommodative strategies of coping. *Psychology and Aging, 5,* 58–67. https://doi.org/10.1037/0882-7974.5.1.58

Brickman, P., Coates, D., & Janoff-Bulman, R. (1978). Lottery winners and accident victims: is happiness relative? *Journal of Personality and Social Psychology, 36,* 917–927. https://doi.org/10.1037/0022-3514.36.8.917

Britton, A., Shipley, M., Singh-Manoux, A., & Marmot, M. G. (2008). Successful aging: the contribution of early-life and midlife risk factors. *Journal of the American Geriatrics Society, 56,* 1098–1105. https://doi.org/10.1111/j.1532-5415.2008.01740.x

Burnes, D., Sheppard, C., Henderson Jr, C. R., Wassel, M., Cope, R., Barber, C., & Pillemer, K. (2019). Interventions to reduce ageism against older adults: a systematic review and meta-analysis. *American Journal of Public Health, 109,* e1–e9. https://doi.org/10.2105/AJPH.2019.305123

Butler, R. N. (1968). The life review: an interpretation of reminiscence in the aged. In B. L. Neugarten (Ed.), *Middle age and aging* (pp. 486–496). The University of Chicago Press.

Calasanti, T. M. (2016). Combating ageism: how successful is successful aging? *The Gerontologist, 56,* 1093–1101. https://doi.org/10.1093/geront/gnv076

Calasanti, T. M., & Slevin, K. F. (2001). *Gender, social inequalities, and aging.* AltaMiraPress.

Calasanti, T. M., & King, N. (2020). Beyond successful aging 2.0: inequalities, ageism, and the case for normalizing old ages. *The Journals of Gerontology Series B: Psychological Sciences and Social Sciences*, gbaa037. https://doi.org/doi:10.1093/geronb/gbaa037

Calasanti, T., King, N., Pietilä, I., & Ojala, H. (2018). Rationales for anti-aging activities in middle Age: aging, health, or appearance? *The Gerontologist*, *58*, 233–241. https://doi.org/10.1093/geront/gnw111

Cannon, W. B. (1929). Organisation for physiological homeostasis. *Physiological Reviews*, *9*, 399–431. https://doi.org/10.1152/physrev.1929.9.3.399

Cannon, W. B. (1939). Aging of homeostatic mechanisms. In E. V. Cowdry (Ed.), *Process of aging: social and psychological perspectives*. (pp. 567–582). Williams and Wilkins.

Carmel, S. (2019). Health and well-being in late life: gender differences worldwide. *Frontiers in Medicine*, *6*, 218. https://doi.org/10.3389/fmed.2019.00218

Charness, N., & Schaie, K. W. (Eds). (2003). *Impact of technology on successful aging*. Springer Publishing Company.

Chiang, K. J., Chu, H., Chang, H. J., Chung, M. H., Chen, C. H., Chiou, H. Y., & Chou, K. R. (2010). The effects of reminiscence therapy on psychological well-being, depression, and loneliness among the institutionalized aged. *International Journal of Geriatric Psychiatry*, *25*, 380–388. https://doi.org/10.1002/gps.2350

Chonody, J. M., & Teater, B. (2016). Why do I dread looking old? A test of social identity theory, terror management theory, and the double standard of aging. *Journal of Women and Aging*, *28*, 112–126. https://doi.org/10.1080/08952841.2014.950533

Clarke, L. H., & Griffin, M. (2008). Visible and invisible ageing: beauty work as a response to ageism. *Ageing and Society*, *28*, 653–674. https://doi.org/10.1017/S0144686X07007003

Cohen, S., Janicki-Deverts, D., Chen, E., & Matthews, K. A. (2010). Childhood socioeconomic status and adult health. *Annals of the New York Academy of Sciences*, *1186*, 37–55. https://doi.org/10.1111/j.1749-6632.2009.05334.x

Collins, T. A., Dumas, T. L., & Moyer, L. P. (2017). Intersecting disadvantages: race, gender, and age discrimination among attorneys. *Social Science Quarterly*, *98*, 1642–1658. https://doi.org/10.1111/ssqu.12376

Cosco, T. D., Prina, A. M., Perales, J., Stephan, B. C., & Brayne, C. (2013). Lay perspectives of successful ageing: a systematic review and meta-ethnography. *BMJ Open*, *3*, e002710. https://doi.org/10.1136/bmjopen-2013-002710

Cottrell, L., & Duggleby, W. (2016). The 'good death': an integrative literature review. *Palliative and Supportive Care*, *14*, 686–712. https://doi.org/10.1017/S1478951515001285

Cowdry, E. V. (Ed.). (1939). *Problems of ageing: biological and medical aspects*. Williams and Wilkins.

Crimmins, E. M. (2021). Recent trends and increasing differences in life expectancy present opportunities for multidisciplinary research on aging. *Nature Aging*, *1*, 12–13. https://doi.org/10.1038/s43587-020-00016-0

Crimmins, E. M., & Beltrán-Sánchez, H. (2011). Mortality and morbidity trends: is there compression of morbidity? *The Journal of Gerontology Series B: Psychological Sciences and Social Sciences*, *66B*, 75–86. https://doi.org/10.1093/geronb/gbq088

Crimmins, E. M., Zhang, Y., & Saito, Y. (2016). Trends over 4 decades in disability-free life expectancy in the United States. *American Journal of Public Health, 106*, 1287–1293. https://doi.org/10.2105/AJPH.2016.303120

Cross, S. H., & Warraich, H. J. (2019). Changes in the place of death in the United States. *New England Journal of Medicine, 381*, 2369–2370. https://doi.org/10.1056/NEJMc1911892

Czaja, S. J., Kallestrup, P., & Harvey, P. D. (2020). Evaluation of a novel technology-based program designed to assess and train everyday skills in older adults. *Innovation in Aging, 4*, 1–10. https://doi.org/10.1093/geroni/igaa052

Czaja, S. J., Boot, W. R., Charness, N., Rogers, W. A., & Sharit, J. (2018). Improving social support for older adults through technology: findings from the PRISM randomized controlled trial. *The Gerontologist, 58*, 467–477. https://doi.org/10.1093/geront/gnw249

Daatland, S. O., & Biggs, S. (2006). *Ageing and diversity: multiple pathways and cultural migrations.* Policy Press.

Dannefer, D. (2003). Cumulative advantage/disadvantage and the life course: cross-fertilizing age and social science theory. *The Journal of Gerontology Series B: Psychological Sciences and Social Sciences, 58B*, S327–S337. https://doi.org/10.1093/geronb/58.6.S327

Dasch, B., Blum, K., Gude, P., & Bausewein, C. (2015). Place of death: trends over the course of a decade: a population-based study of death certificates from the years 2001 and 2011. *Deutsches Ärzteblatt International, 112*, 496–504. https://doi.org/10.3238/arztebl.2015.0496

Daskalopoulou, C., Stubbs, B., Kralj, C., Koukounari, A., Prince, M., & Prina, A. M. (2017). Physical activity and healthy ageing: a systematic review and meta-analysis of longitudinal cohort studies. *Ageing Research Reviews, 38*, 6–17. https://doi.org/10.1016/j.arr.2017.06.00

de Labra, C., Guimaraes-Pinheiro, C., Maseda, A., Lorenzo, T., & Millán-Calenti, J. C. (2015). Effects of physical exercise interventions in frail older adults: a systematic review of randomized controlled trials. *BMC Geriatrics, 15*, 154. https://doi.org/10.1186/s12877-015-0155-4

De Roo, M. L., Miccinesi, G., Onwuteaka-Philipsen, B. D., Van Den Noortgate, N., Van den Block, L., Bonacchi, A., Donker, G. A., Alonso, J. E. L., Moreels, S., Deliens, L., & Francke, A. L. (2014). Actual and preferred place of death of home-dwelling patients in four European countries: making sense of quality indicators. *PLoS ONE, 9*, e93762. https://doi.org/10.1371/journal.pone.0093762

de São José, J. M., Timonen, V., Amado, C. A. F., & Santos, S. P. (2017). A critique of the Active Ageing Index. *Journal of Aging Studies, 40*, 49–56. https://doi.org/10.1016/j.jaging.2017.01.001

Deary, I. J., Whiteman, M. C., Starr, J. M., Whalley, L. J., & Fox, H. C. (2004). The impact of childhood intelligence on later life: following up the Scottish mental surveys of 1932 and 1947. *Journal of Personality and Social Psychology, 86*, 130. https://doi.org/DOI:10.1037/0022-3514.86.1.130

Demetrius, L., & Legendre, S. (2013). Evolutionary entropy predicts the outcome of selection: competition for resources that vary in abundance and diversity. *Theoretical Population Biology, 83*, 39–54. https://doi.org/10.1016/j.tpb.2012.10.004

Demirovic, D., & Rattan, S. I. S. (2013). Establishing cellular stress response profiles as biomarkers of homeodynamics, health and hormesis. *Experimental Gerontology*, *48*, 94–98. https://doi.org/10.1016/j.exger.2012.02.005

Depp, C. A., & Jeste, D. V. (2006). Definitions and predictors of successful aging: a comprehensive review of larger quantitative studies. *The American Journal of Geriatric Psychiatry*, *14*, 6–20. https://doi.org/10.1097/01.JGP.0000192501.03069.bc

Dewey, J. (1931). The development of American pragmatism. In J. Dewy (Ed.), Philosophy and civilization (pp. 13–35). G.P. Puntnam's Sons.

Diehl, M., & Wahl, H.-W. (2020). *The psychology of later life: a contextual perspective*. American Psychological Association Books. https://doi.org/doi:10.1037/0000185-000

Diener, E. (2000). Subjective well-being: the science of happiness and a proposal for a national index. *American Psychologist*, *55*, 34–43. https://doi.org/10.1037/0003-066X.55.1.34

Diener, E., Lucas, R. E., & Scollon, C. N. (2006). Beyond the hedonic treadmill: revising the adaptation theory of well-being. *American Psychologist*, *61*, 305–314. https://doi.org/10.1037/0003-066X.61.4.305

Diener, E., Lucas, R., Schimmack, U., & Helliwell, J. F. (2009). *Well-being for public policy*. Oxford University Press. https://doi.org/10.1093/acprof:oso/9780195334074.001.0001

Dilli, S., Carmichael, S. G., & Rijpma, A. (2019). Introducing the historical gender equality index. *Feminist Economics*, *25*, 31–57. https://doi.org/10.1080/13545701.2018.1442582

Dixon, J., King, D., & Knapp, M. (2019). Advance care planning in England: is there an association with place of death? Secondary analysis of data from the National Survey of Bereaved People. *BMJ Supportive & Palliative Care*, *9*, 316–325. https://doi.org/10.1136/bmjspcare-2015-000971

Dobbs, D., Eckert, J. K., Rubinstein, B., Keimig, L., Clark, L., Frankowski, A. C., & Zimmerman, S. (2008). An ethnographic study of stigma and ageism in residential care or assisted living. *The Gerontologist*, *48*, 517–526, https://doi.org/10.1093/geront/48.4.517

Dugravot, A., Fayosse, A., Dumurgier, J., Bouillon, K., Rayana, T. B., Schnitzler, A., Kivimaki, M., Sabia, S., & Singh-Manoux, A. (2020). Social inequalities in multimorbidity, frailty, disability, and transitions to mortality: a 24-year follow-up of the Whitehall II cohort study. *The Lancet Public Health*, *5*, e42–e50. https://doi.org/10.1016/S2468-2667(19)30226-9

Ehni, H.-J., & Wahl, H.-W. (2020). Six propositions against ageism in the COVID-19 pandemic. *Journal of Aging & Social Policy*, *32*, 515–525. https://doi.org/10.1080/08959420.2020.17700321

Eibich, P., Krekel, C., Demuth, I., & Wagner, G. G. (2016). Associations between neighborhood characteristics, well-being and health vary over the life course. *Gerontology*, *62*, 362–370. https://doi.org/10.1159/000438700

Eikemo, T. A., & Bambra, C. (2008). The welfare state: a glossary for public health. *Journal of Epidemiology & Community Health*, *62*, 3–6. https://doi.org/10.1136/jech.2007.066787

Erikson, E. H. (1963). *Childhood and society* (2nd rev. ed.). Norton

Erikson, E. H. (1968). *Identity. Youth and crisis.* Norton.

Erikson, E. H. (1982). *The life cycle completed.* Norton.

Erikson, E. H., & Erikson, J. M. (1997). *The life cycle completed.* Norton.

Esping-Andersen, G. (Ed.). (1990). *Three worlds of welfare capitalism.* Polity Press.

Fabbre, V. D. (2015). Gender transitions in later life: a queer perspective on successful aging. *The Gerontologist, 55,* 144–153. https://doi.org/10.1093/geront/gnu079

Ferraro, K. F., & Shippee, T. P. (2009). Aging and cumulative inequality: how does inequality get under the skin? *The Gerontologist, 49,* 333–343. https://doi.org/10.1093/geront/gnp034

Ferraro, K. F., Schafer, M. H., & Wilkinson, L. R. (2016). Childhood disadvantage and health problems in middle and later life: early imprints on physical health? *American Sociological Review, 81,* 107–133. https://doi.org/10.1177/0003122415619617

Ferraro, K. F., Kemp, B. R., & Williams, M. M. (2017). Diverse aging and health inequality by race and ethnicity. *Innovation in Aging, 1,* igx0021. https://doi.org/10.1093/geroni/igx002

Finch, C. E. (2009). Update on slow aging and negligible senescence—a mini-review. *Gerontology, 55,* 307–313. https://doi.org/10.1159/000215589

Finch, C. E., & Kirkwood, T. B. L. (2000). *Chance, development, and aging.* Oxford University Press.

Finlay, R. (1978). The Venetian republic as a gerontocracy: age and politics in the renaissance. *Journal of Medieval and Renaissance Studies, 8,* 157–178. https://doi.org/10.1007/978-3-319-69892-2_820-1

Fitzgerald, K. G., & Caro, F. G. (2014). An overview of age-friendly cities and communities around the world. *Journal of Aging & Social Policy, 26,* 1–18. https://doi.org/10.1080/08959420.2014.860786

Fontana, L., & Partridge, L. (2015). Promoting health and longevity through diet: from model organisms to humans. *Cell, 161,* 106–118. https://doi.org/10.1016/j.cell.2015.02.020

Fortin, M., Hudon, C., Haggerty, J., van den Akker, M., & Almirall, J. (2010). Prevalence estimates of multimorbidity: a comparative study of two sources. *BMC Health Services Research, 10,* 111. https://doi.org/10.1186/1472-6963-10-111

Foster, L., & Walker, A. (2015). Active and successful aging: a European policy perspective. *The Gerontologist, 55,* 83–90. https://doi.org/10.1093/geront/gnu028

Fries, J. F. (1980). Aging, natural death, and the compression of morbidity. *The New England Journal of Medicine, 303,* 130–135. https://doi.org/10.1056/NEJM198007173030304

Fries, J. F., Bruce, B., & Chakravarty, E. (2011). Compression of morbidity 1980–2011: a focused review of paradigms and progress. *Journal of Aging Research, 2011,* 261702. https://doi.org/10.4061/2011/261702

Fulop, T., Larbi, A., Witkowski, J. M., McElhaney, J., Loeb, M., Mitnitski, A., & Pawelec, G. (2010). Aging, frailty and age-related diseases. *Biogerontology, 11,* 547–563. https://doi.org/10.1007/s10522-010-9287-2

Gao, X., Zhang, W., Wang, Y., Pedram, P., Cahill, F., Zhai, G., Randell, E., Gulliver, W., & Sun, G. (2016). Serum metabolic biomarkers distinguish metabolically healthy peripherally obese from unhealthy centrally obese individuals. *Nutrition & Metabolism, 13*, 33. https://doi.org/10.1186/s12986-016-0095-9

Gatz, M., & Zarit, S. H. (1999). A good old age: paradox or possibility. In V. L. Bengtson & K. W. Schaie (Eds), *Handbook of theories of aging* (pp. 396–416). Springer.

Geissler, B., & Pfau-Effinger, B. (2005). Change in European care arrangements. In B. Pfau-Effinger & B. Geissler (Eds), *Care and social integration in European societies* (pp. 3–19). Policy Press.

George, L. K. (2010). Still happy after all these years: research frontiers on subjective well-being in later life. *The Journal of Gerontology Series B: Psychological Sciences and Social Sciences, 65B*, 331–339. https://doi.org/10.1093/geronb/gbq006

Gerstorf, D., & Ram, N. (2015). A framework for studying mechanisms underlying terminal decline in well-being. *International Journal of Behavioral Development, 39*, 210–220. https://doi.org/10.1177/0165025414565408

Gerstorf, D., Ram, N., Estabrook, R., Schupp, J., Wagner, G. G., & Lindenberger, U. (2008). Life satisfaction shows terminal decline in old age: longitudinal evidence from the German Socio-Economic Panel Study (SOEP). *Developmental Psychology, 44*, 1148–1159. https://doi.org/10.1037/0012-1649.44.4.1148

Gerstorf, D., Ram, N., Mayraz, G., Hidajat, M., Lindenberger, U., Wagner, G. G., & Schupp, J. (2010a). Late-life decline in well-being across adulthood in Germany, the United Kingdom, and the United States: something is seriously wrong at the end of life. *Psychology And Aging, 25*, 477–485. https://doi.org/10.1037/a0017543

Gerstorf, D., Ram, N., Goebel, J., Schupp, J., Lindenberger, U., & Wagner, G. G. (2010b). Where people live and die makes a difference: individual and geographic disparities in well-being progression at the end of life. *Psychology and Aging, 25*, 661–676. https://doi.org/10.1037/a0019574

Gerstorf, D., Hoppmann, C. A., Löckenhoff, C. E., Infurna, F. J., Schupp, J., Wagner, G. G., & Ram, N. (2016). Terminal decline in well-being: the role of social orientation. *Psychology And Aging, 31*, 149–165. https://doi.org/10.1037/pag0000072

Gewirtz-Meydan, A., & Ayalon, L. (2018). Forever young: visual representations of gender and age in online dating sites for older adults. *Journal of Women & Aging, 30*, 484–502. https://doi.org/10.1080/08952841.2017.1330586

Gignac, M. A., Cott, C., & Badley, E. M. (2000). Adaptation to chronic illness and disability and its relationship to perceptions of independence and dependence. *The Journal of Gerontology Series B: Psychological Sciences and Social Sciences, 55*, P362–P372. https://doi.org/10.1093/geronb/55.6.P362

Gilligan, C. (1982). *In a different voice*. Harvard University Press.

Goldberg, D. S. (2012). Social justice, health inequalities and methodological individualism in US health promotion. *Public Health Ethics, 5*, 104–115. https://doi.org/10.1093/phe/phs013

Gomes, B., Calanzani, N., & Higginson, I. J. (2011). *Local preferences and place of death in regions within England 2010*. Cicely Saunders International.

Gott, M., & Ingleton, C. (2011). *Living with ageing and dying: palliative and end of life care for older people*. Oxford University Press.

Greenfield, E. A., Black, K., Buffel, T., & Yeh, J. (2019). Community gerontology: a framework for research, policy, and practice on communities and aging. *The Gerontologist, 59*, 803–810. https://doi.org/10.1093/geront/gny089

Gruman, G. J. (1966). A history of ideas about the prolongation of life: the evolution of prolongevity hypotheses to 1800. *Transactions of the American Philosophical Society, 56*, 1–102. http://hdl.handle.net/10822/762562

Haase, C. M., Heckhausen, J., & Wrosch, C. (2013). Developmental regulation across the life span: toward a new synthesis. *Developmental Psychology, 49*, 964–972. https://doi.org/10.1037/a0029231

Haber, C. (2004). Life extension and history: the continual search for the fountain of youth. *The Journal of Gerontology Series A: Biological Sciences and Medical Sciences, 59*, B515–B522. https://doi.org/10.1093/gerona/59.6.B515

Hakim, A. B. (2016). *Historical introduction to philosophy*. Routledge.

Hank, K. (2011). How 'successful' do older Europeans age? Findings from SHARE. *The Journal of Gerontology, Series B: Psychological Sciences and Social Sciences, 66B*, 230–236. https://doi.org/10.1093/geronb/gbq089

Harper, S. (2014). Economic and social implications of aging societies. *Science, 346*, 587–591. https://doi.org/10.1126/science.1254405

Havighurst, R. J. (1961). Successful aging. *The Gerontologist, 1*, 8–13. https://doi.org/10.1093/geront/1.1.8

Havighurst, R. J. (1963). Successful aging. In R. H. Williams, C. Tibbits, & W. Donanue (Eds), *Processes of aging: social and psychological perspectives* (pp. 299–320). Atherton Press.

Havighurst, R. J., & Albrecht, R. (1953). *Older people*. Longmans, Green and Co.

Hayflick, L. (2007). Entropy explains aging, genetic determinism explains longevity, and undefined terminology explains misunderstanding both. *PLoS Genetics, 3*, e220. https://doi.org/doi:10.1371/journal.pgen.0030220

Heckhausen, J., & Buchmann, M. (2019). A multi-disciplinary model of life-course canalization and agency. *Advances in Life Course Research, 41*, 100246. https://doi.org/10.1016/j.alcr.2018.09.002

Heckhausen, J., & Schulz, R. (1993). Optimisation by selection and compensation: balancing primary and secondary control in life span development. *International Journal of Behavioral Development, 16*, 287–303. https://doi.org/10.1177/016502549301600210

Hellström, I., Håkanson, C., Eriksson, H., & Sandberg, J. (2017). Development of older men's caregiving roles for wives with dementia. *Scandinavian Journal of Caring Sciences, 31*, 957–964. https://doi.org/10.1111/scs.12419

Herd, P. (2006). Do functional health inequalities decrease in old age? Educational status and functional decline among the 1931–1941 birth cohort. *Research on Aging, 28*, 375–392. https://doi.org/10.1177/0164027505285845

Hertzog, C. (2009). Use it or lose it: an old hypothesis, new evidence, and an ongoing case study. In H. B. Bosworth & C. Hertzog (Eds), *Decade of behavior (2000–2010). Aging and cognition: research methodologies and empirical advances* (pp. 161–179). American Psychological Association. https://doi.org/10.1037/11882-008

Higgs, P., & Gilleard, C. (2020). The ideology of ageism versus the social imaginary of the fourth age: two differing approaches to the negative contexts of old age. *Ageing and Society, 40*, 1617–1630. https://doi.org/10.1017/S0144686X19000096

Hinterlong, J. E., Morrow-Howell, N., & Rozario, P. A. (2007). Productive engagement and late life physical and mental health: findings from a nationally representative panel study. *Research on Aging, 29*, 348–370. https://doi.org/10.1177/0164027507300806

Holliday, R. (2007). *Ageing: the paradox of life.* Springer.

Hoppmann, C. A., & Gerstorf, D. (2016). Social interrelations in aging: the sample case of married couples. In K. W. Schaie, S. L. Willis, B. G. Knight, B. Levy, & D. C. Park (Eds), *Handbook of the psychology of aging* (8th ed., pp. 263–277). Academic Press. https://doi.org/10.1016/B978-0-12-411469-2.00014-5

House, J. S., Lantz, P. M., & Herd, P. (2005). Continuity and change in the social stratification of aging and health over the life course: evidence from a nationally representative longitudinal study from 1986 to 2001/2002 (Americans' Changing Lives Study). *The Journal of Gerontology Series B: Psychological Sciences and Social Sciences, 60*(Special Issue 2), S15–S26. https://doi.org/10.1093/geronb/60.Special_Issue_2.S15

Hu, Y., Leinonen, T., Myrskylä, M., & Martikainen, P. (2020). Changes in socioeconomic differences in hospital days with age: cumulative disadvantage, age-as-leveler, or both? *The Journal of Gerontology: Series B: Psychological Sciences and Social Sciences, 75*, 1336–1347. https://doi.org/10.1093/geronb/gbx161

Hursthouse, R., & Pettigrove, G. (2018). Virtue ethics. In E. N. Zalta (Ed.), *The Stanford Encyclopedia of Philosophy.* Stanford University. https://plato.stanford.edu/archives/win2018/entries/ethics-virtue

Iwarsson, S. (2004). Assessing the fit between older people and their physical home environments: an occupational therapy research perspective. *Annual Review of Gerontology and Geriatrics, 23*, 85–109.

Iwarsson, S., Wahl, H.-W., Nygren, C., Oswald, F., Sixsmith, A., Sixsmith, J., Széman, Z., & Tomsone, S. (2007). Importance of the home environment for healthy aging: conceptual and methodological background of the European ENABLE-AGE Project. *The Gerontologist, 47*, 78–84. https://doi.org/10.1093/geront/47.1.78

Jagger, C., Gillies, C., Moscone, F., Cambois, E., Van Oyen, H., Nusselder, W., & Robine, J.-M. (2008). Inequalities in healthy life years in the 25 countries of the European Union in 2005: a cross-national meta-regression analysis. *Lancet, 372*, 2124–2131. https://doi.org/10.1016/S0140-6736(08)61594-9

Jazwinski, S. M. (1998). Genetics of longevity. *Experimental Gerontology, 33*, 773–783. https://doi.org/10.1016/S0531-5565(98)00027-8

Jeong, S. Y. S., Higgins, I., & McMillan, M. (2010). The essentials of Advance Care Planning for end-of-life care for older people. *Journal of Clinical Nursing, 19*, 389–397. https://doi.org/10.1111/j.1365-2702.2009.03001.x

Jönson, H. (2013). We will be vifferent! Ageism and the temporal construction of old age. *The Gerontologist, 53*, 198–204. https://doi.org/10.1093/geront/gns066

Jopp, D. S., Wozniak, D., Damarin, A. K., De Feo, M., Jung, S., & Jeswani, S. (2015). How could lay perspectives on successful aging complement scientific theory? Findings from a U.S. and a German life-span sample. *The Gerontologist, 55*, 91–106. https://doi.org/10.1093/geront/gnu059

Kahn, R. L., & Antonucci, T. C. (1980). Convoys over the life course: attachment, roles and social support. In P. B. Baltes & O. G. Brim, Jr. (Eds), *Life-span development and behavior* (Vol. 3, pp. 253–286). Academic Press.

Kamin, S. T., & Lang, F. R. (2020). Internet use and cognitive functioning in late adult-hood: longitudinal findings from the Survey of Health, Ageing and Retirement in Europe (SHARE). *The Journal of Gerontology Series B: Psychological Sciences and Social Sciences, 75*, 534–539. https://doi.org/10.1093/geronb/gby123

Kane, R. A. (2001). Long-term care and a good quality of life: bringing them closer together. *The Gerontologist, 41*, 293–304. https://doi.org/10.1093/geront/41.3.293

Katz, S. (2001). Growing older without aging? Positive aging, anti-ageism, and anti-aging. *Generations: Journal of the American Society on Aging, 25*, 27–32. https://doi.org/10.2307/26555099

Katz, S., & Calasanti, T. (2015). Critical perspectives on successful aging: does it 'appeal more than it illuminates'? *The Gerontologist, 55*, 26–33. https://doi.org/doi:10.1093/geront/gnu027

Kessler, E.-M., & Staudinger, U. M. (2007). Intergenerational potential: effects of so-cial interaction between older adults and adolescents. *Psychology And Aging, 22*, 690–704. https://doi.org/10.1037/0882-7974.22.4.690

King, H. (1986). Tithonos and the Tettix. *Arethusa, 19*, 15–35.

Kivnick, H. Q., & Wells, C. K. (2014). Untapped richness in Erik H. Erikson's root-stock. *The Gerontologist, 54*, 40–50. https://doi.org/10.1093/geront/gnt123

Klatz, R., & Goldman, R. M. (1997). *Anti-age medical therapeutics*. Health Quest Publications.

Koenig, H. G., McCullough, M. E., & Larson, D. B. (Eds). (2001). *Handbook of religion and health*. Oxford University Press.

Kotter-Grühn, D., Kleinspehn-Ammerlahn, A., Gerstorf, D., & Smith, J. (2009). Self-perceptions of aging predict mortality and change with approaching death: 16-year longitudinal results from the Berlin Aging Study. *Psychology And Aging, 24*, 654–667. https://doi.org/10.1037/a0016510

Krause, N. (2006). Religion and health in late life. In J. E. Birren & W. K. Schaie (Eds), *Handbook of the psychology of aging* (pp. 499–518). Elsevier Academic Press. https://doi.org/10.1016/B978-012101264-9/50025-2

Krekula, C., Nikander, P., & Wilińska, M. (2018). Multiple marginalizations based on age: gendered ageism and beyond. In L. Ayalon & C. Tesch-Römer (Eds), *Contemporary perspectives on ageism* (pp. 33–50). Springer. https://doi.org/10.1007/978-3-319-73820-8_3

Kunzmann, U., Little, T. D., & Smith, J. (2000). Is age-related stability of subjective well-being a paradox? Cross-sectional and longitudional evidence from the Berlin Aging Study. *Psychology and Aging, 15*, 511–526. https://doi.org/10.1037/0882-7974.15.3.511

Lachman, V. D. (2012). Applying the ethics of care to your nursing practice. *Medsurg Nursing, 21*, 112–116.

Lampe, K. (2015). *The birth of hedonism: the Cyrenaic philosophers and pleasure as a way of life*. Princeton University Press.

Lawton, M. P. (1989). Environmental proactivity in older people. In V. L. Bengtson & K. W. Schaie (Eds), *The course of later life* (pp. 15–23). Springer.

Lawton, M. P., & Nahemow, L. (1973). Ecology and the aging process. In C. Eisdorfer & M. P. Lawton (Eds), *The psychology of adult development and aging* (pp. 619–674). American Psychological Association. https://doi.org/10.1037/10044-020

Lawton, M. P., & Simon, B. (1968). The ecology of social relationships in housing for the elderly. *The Gerontologist, 8,* 108–115. https://doi.org/10.1093/geront/8.2.108

Lee, H. R., & Riek, L. D. (2018). Reframing assistive robots to promote successful aging. *ACM Transactions on Human-Robot Interaction (THRI), 7,* 1–23. https://doi.org/10.1145/3203303

Leon, D. A. (2011). Trends in European life expectancy: a salutary view. *International Journal of Epidemiology, 40,* 271–277. https://doi.org/10.1093/ije/dyr061

Levy, B. (2009). Stereotype embodiment: a psychosocial approach to aging. *Current Directions in Psychological Science, 18,* 332–336. https://doi.org/10.1111/j.1467-8721.2009.01662.x

Levy, B. R., & Myers, L. M. (2004). Preventive health behaviors influenced by self-perceptions of aging. *Preventive Medicine, 39,* 625–629. https://doi.org/10.1016/j.ypmed.2004.02.029

Levy, B. R., Slade, M. D., Chang, E.-S., Kannoth, S., & Wang, S.-Y. (2020). Ageism amplifies cost and prevalence of health conditions. *The Gerontologist, 60,* 174–181. https://doi.org/10.1093/geront/gny131

Lewer, D., Jayatunga, W., Aldridge, R. W., Edge, C., Marmot, M., Story, A., & Hayward, A. (2020). Premature mortality attributable to socioeconomic inequality in England between 2003 and 2018: an observational study. *The Lancet Public Health, 5,* e33–e41. https://doi.org/10.1016/S2468-2667(19)30219-1

Liang, J., & Luo, B. (2012). Toward a discourse shift in social gerontology: from successful aging to harmonious aging. *Journal of Aging Studies, 26,* 327–334. https://doi.org/10.1016/j.jaging.2012.03.001

Lindenberger, U., Lövdén, M., Schellenbach, M., Li, S.-C., & Krüger, A. (2008). Psychological principles of successful aging technologies: a mini-review. *Gerontology, 54,* 59–68. https://doi.org/10.1159/000116114

Löckenhoff, C. E., & Carstensen, L. L. (2004). Socioemotional selectivity theory, aging, and health: the increasingly delicate balance between regulating emotions and making tough choices. *Journal of Personality, 72,* 1395–1424. https://doi.org/10.1111/j.1467-6494.2004.00301.x

Loos, E., & Ivan, L. (2018). Visual ageism in the media. In L. Ayalon & C. Tesch-Römer (Eds), *Contemporary perspectives on ageism* (pp. 163–176). Springer. https://doi.org/10.1007/978-3-319-73820-8_11

López-Otín, C., Blasco, M. A., Partridge, L., Serrano, M., & Kroemer, G. (2013). The hallmarks of aging. *Cell, 153,* 1194–1217. https://doi.org/10.1016/j.cell.2013.05.039

Lorenzo-López, L., Maseda, A., de Labra, C., Regueiro-Folgueira, L., Rodríguez-Villamil, J. L., & Millán-Calenti, J. C. (2017). Nutritional determinants of frailty in older adults: a systematic review. *BMC Geriatrics, 17,* 108. https://doi.org/10.1186/s12877-017-0496-2

Lowry, K. A., Vallejo, A. N., & Studenski, S. A. (2012). Successful aging as a continuum of functional independence: lessons from physical disability models of aging. *Aging and Disease, 3,* 5–15.

Luhmann, M., & Intelisano, S. (2018). Hedonic adaptation and the set point for subjective well-being. In E. Diener, S. Oishi, & L. Tay (Eds), *Handbook of well-being.* DEF Publishers. https://doi.org/nobascholar.com

Lyons, A., Alba, B., Heywood, W., Fileborn, B., Minichiello, V., Barrett, C., Hinchliff, S., Malta, S., & Dow, B. (2018). Experiences of ageism and the mental health of older adults. *Aging & Mental Health*, *22*, 1456–1464. https://doi.org/10.1080/ 13607863.2017.1364347

Maddox, G. L. (1987). Aging differently. *The Gerontologist*, *27*, 557–564. https:// doi.org/10.1093/geront/27.5.557

Marquardt, G., Bueter, K., & Motzek, T. (2014). Impact of the design of the built environment on people with dementia: an evidence-based review. *HERD: Health Environments Research & Design Journal*, *8*, 127–157. https://doi.org/10.1177/ 193758671400800111

McAdams, K. K., Lucas, R. E., & Donnellan, M. B. (2012). The role of domain satisfaction in explaining the paradoxical association between life satisfaction and age. *Social Indicators Research*, *109*, 295–303. https://doi.org/10.1007/ s11205-011-9903-9

McGann, M., Ong, R., Bowman, D., Duncan, A., Kimberley, H., & Biggs, S. (2016). Gendered ageism in Australia: changing perceptions of age discrimination among older men and women. *Economic Papers*, *35*, 375–388. https://doi.org/10.1111/ 1759-3441.12155

McLaughlin, S. J., Connell, C. M., Heeringa, S. G., Li, L. W., & Roberts, J. S. (2010). Successful aging in the United States: prevalence estimates from a national sample of older adults. *The Journal of Gerontology Series B: Psychological Sciences and Social Sciences*, *65B*, 216–226. https://doi.org/10.1093/geronb/gbp101

Meier, E. A., Gallegos, J. V., Montross-Thomas, L. P., Depp, C. A., Irwin, S. A., & Jeste, D. V. (2016). Defining a good death (successful dying): literature review and a call for research and public dialogue. *The American Journal of Geriatric Psychiatry*, *24*, 261–271. https://doi.org/10.1016/j.jagp.2016.01.135

Mendes de Leon, C. F., Cagney, K. A., Bienias, J. L., Barnes, L. L., Skarupski, K. A., Scherr, P. A., & Evans, D. A. (2009). Neighborhood social cohesion and disorder in relation to walking in community-dwelling older adults: a multilevel analysis. *Journal of Aging and Health*, *21*, 155–171. https://doi.org/10.1177/ 0898264308328650

Minichiello, V., Browne, J., & Kendig, H. (2000). Perceptions and consequences of ageism: views of older people. *Ageing and Society*, *20*, 253–278. https://doi.org/ 10.1017/S0144686X99007710

Mitnitski, A., Howlett, S. E., & Rockwood, K. (2017). Heterogeneity of human aging and its assessment. *The Journal of Gerontology Series A: Biomedical Sciences and Medical Sciences*, *72*, 877–884. https://doi.org/https://doi.org/10.1093/gerona/ glw089

Nascher, I. L. (1910). Pathology in old age. *Medical Council*, *15*, 94–99.

Nelson, E. A., & Dannefer, D. (1992). Aged heterogeneity: fact or fiction? The fate of diversity in gerontological research. *The Gerontologist*, *32*, 17–23. https://doi.org/ 10.1093/geront/32.1.17

Neugarten, B. L. (1974). Age groups in American society and the rise of the young-old. *The Annals of the American Academy of Political and Social Sciences*, *415*, 187–198. https://doi.org/10.1177/000271627441500114

Neugarten, B. L., Havighurst, R. J., & Tobin, S. S. (1961). The measurement of life satisfaction. *Journal of Gerontoloy, 16*, 134–143. https://doi.org/10.1093/geronj/16.2.134

Neumark, D., Burn, I., Button, P., & Chehras, N. (2019). Do state laws protecting older workers from discrimination reduce age discrimination in hiring? Evidence from a field experiment. *The Journal of Law and Economics, 62*, 373–402. https://doi.org/10.1086/704008

Nicholson, D. J. (2019). Is the cell really a machine? *Journal of Theoretical Biology, 477*, 108–126. https://doi.org/10.1016/j.jtbi.2019.06.002

Oishi, S., Diener, E., Lucas, R. E., & Suh, E. M. (2009). Cross-cultural variations in predictors of life satisfaction: perspectives from needs and values. In E. Diener (Ed.), *Culture and well-being* (pp. 109–127). Springer.

Olshansky, S. J., Perry, D., Miller, R. A., & Butler, R. N. (2007). Pursuing the longevity dividend: scientific goals for an aging world. *Annals of the New York Academy of Sciences, 1114*, 11–13. https://doi.org/10.1196/annals.1396.050

O'Rand, A. M. (2016). Long, broad, and deep. Theoretical approaches in aging and inequality. In V. L. Bengtson, R. A. Settersten, B. K. Kennedy, N. Morrow-Howell, & J. Smith (Eds), *Handbook of theories of aging* (3rd ed., pp. 365–379). Springer.

Orem, D. E., & Taylor, S. G. (2011). Reflections on nursing practice science: the nature, the structure, and the foundation of nursing sciences. *Nursing Science Quarterly, 24*, 35–41. https://doi.org/10.1177/0894318410389061

Oswald, F., & Wahl, H.-W. (2005). Dimensions of the meaning of home in later life. In G. D. Rowles & H. Chaudhury (Eds), *Home and identity in late life: international perspectives* (pp. 21–45). Springer.

Oswald, F., Wahl, H.-W., Schilling, O., Nygren, C., Fänge, A., Sixsmith, A., Sixsmith, J., Szeman, Z., Tomsone, S., & Iwarsson, S. (2007). Relationships between housing and healthy aging in very old age. *The Gerontologist, 47*, 96–107. https://doi.org/10.1093/geront/47.1.96

Pasupathi, M., & Carstensen, L. L. (2003). Age and emotional expericence during mutual reminiscing. *Psychology And Aging, 18*, 430–442. https://doi.org/10.1037/0882-7974.18.3.430

Paterson, J. G., & Zderad, L. T. (1976). *Humanistic Nursing*. National League for Nursing

Peplau, H. E. (1997). Peplau's theory of interpersonal relations. *Nursing Science Quarterly, 10*(4), 162–167. https://doi.org/10.1177/089431849701000407

Permanyer, I. (2013). A critical assessment of the UNDP's gender inequality index. *Feminist Economics, 19*, 1–32. https://doi.org/10.1080/13545701.2013.769687

Petrov, I. C. (2007). The elderly in a period of transition—health, personality, and social aspects of adaptation. *Annals of the New York Academy of Sciences, 1114*, 300–309. https://doi.org/10.1196/annals.1396.041

Pillemer, K., Fuller-Rowell, T. E., Reid, M., & Wells, N. M. (2010). Environmental volunteering and health outcomes over a 20-year period. *The Gerontologist, 50*, 594–602. https://doi.org/10.1093/geront/gnq007

Pinquart, M., & Sörensen, S. (2000). Influences of socioeconomic status, social network, and competence on subjective well-being in later life: a meta-analysis. *Psychology and Aging, 15*, 187–224. https://doi.org/10.1037/0882-7974.15.2.187

Pinquart, M., & Sörensen, S. (2001). Gender differences in self-concept and psychological well-being in old age: a meta-analysis. *Journals of Gerontology: Psychological Sciences, 56B*, P195–P213. https://doi.org/10.1093/geronb/56.4.P195

Präg, P., Wittek, R., & Mills, M. C. (2017). The educational gradient in self-rated health in Europe: does the doctor–patient relationship make a difference? *Acta Sociologica, 60*, 325–341. https://doi.org/10.1177/0001699316670715

Pruchno, R. (2015). Successful aging: contentious past, productive future. *The Gerontologist, 55*, 1–4. https://doi.org/10.1093/geront/gnv002

Rattan, S. I. S. (1995). Gerontogenes: real or virtual? *The FASEB Journal, 9*, 284–286. https://doi.org/10.1096/fasebj.9.2.7781932

Rattan, S. I. S. (1998). The nature of gerontogenes and vitagenes. Antiaging effects of repeated heat shock on human fibroblasts. *Annals of the New York Academy of Sciences, 854*, 54–60. https://doi.org/10.1111/j.1749-6632.1998.tb09891.x

Rattan, S. I. S. (2000). Biogerontology: the next step. *Annals of the New York Academy of Sciences, 908*, 282–290. https://doi.org/10.1111/j.1749-6632.2000.tb06655.x

Rattan, S. I. S. (2006). Theories of biological aging: genes, proteins and free radicals. *Free Radical Research, 40*, 1230–1238. https://doi.org/10.1080/10715760600911303

Rattan, S. I. S. (2008). Increased molecular damage and heterogeneity as the basis of aging. *Biological Chemistry, 389*, 267–272. https://doi.org/10.1515/BC.2008.030

Rattan, S. I. S. (2014). Molecular gerontology: from homeodynamics to hormesis. *Curr Pharm Des, 20*, 3036–3039. https://doi.org/10.2174/13816128113196660708

Rattan, S. I. S. (2015). Biology of ageing: principles, challenges and perspectives. *Romanian Journal of Morphology and Embryology, 56*, 1251–1253. http://www.ncbi.nlm.nih.gov/pubmed/26743268

Rattan, S. I. S. (2020a). Biological health and homeodynamic space. In J. Sholl & S. I. S. Rattan (Eds), *Expaning Health Across the Sciences.* (pp. 43–51). Springer Nature.

Rattan, S. I. S. (2020b). Naive extrapolations, overhyped claims and empty promises in ageing research and interventions need avoidance. *Biogerontology, 21*, 415–421. https://doi.org/10.1007/s10522-019-09851-0

Rescher, N. (1999). *Realistic pragmatism: an introduction to pragmatic philosophy.* SUNY Press.

Riley, M. W. (1998). Successful aging. *The Gerontologist, 38*, 151. https://doi.org/10.1093/geront/38.2.151

Riley, M. W., & Riley, J. W., Jr. (2000). Age integration. Conceptual and historical background. *The Gerontologist, 40*, 266–270. https://doi.org/10.1093/geront/40.3.266

Robert, S. A., & Ruel, E. (2006). Racial segregation and health disparities between black and white older adults. *The Journal of Gerontology Series B: Psychological Sciences and Social Sciences, 61*, S203–S211. https://doi.org/10.1093/geronb/61.4.S203

Rolfson, D. (2018). Successful aging and frailty: a systematic review. *Geriatrics, 3*, 79. https://doi.org/10.3390/geriatrics3040079

Rook, K. S. (2015). Social networks in later life: weighing positive and negative effects on health and well-being. *Current Directions in Psychological Science, 24*, 45–51. https://doi.org/10.1177/0963721414551364

Rowe, J. W., & Carr, D. C. (2018). Successful aging: history and prospects. In O. Braddick (Ed.), *Oxford Research Encyclopedia of Psychology*. Oxford University Press. https://doi.org/10.1093/acrefore/9780190236557.013.342

Rowe, J. W., & Kahn, R. L. (1987). Human aging: usual and successful. *Science, 237*, 143–149. https://doi.org/10.1126/science.3299702

Rowe, J. W., & Kahn, R. L. (1997). Successful aging. *The Gerontologist, 37*, 433–440. https://doi.org/10.1093/geront/37.4.433

Rowe, J. W., & Kahn, R. L. (1998). *Successful aging*. Pantheon Books.

Rowe, J. W., & Kahn, R. L. (2015). Successful aging 2.0: conceptual expansions for the 21st century. *The Journals of Gerontology Series B: Psychological Sciences and Social Sciences, 70*, 593–596. https://doi.org/10.1093/geronb/gbv025

Roy, C. (2011). Extending the Roy adaptation model to meet changing global needs. *Nursing Science Quarterly, 24*, 345–351. https://doi.org/10.1177/0894318411419210

Ryff, C. D. (1982). Successful aging: a developmental approach. *The Gerontologist, 22*, 209–214. https://doi.org/10.1093/geront/22.2.209

Ryff, C. D. (1989). Beyond Ponce de Leon and life satisfaction: new directions in quest of successful ageing. *International Journal of Behavioral Development, 12*, 35–55. https://doi.org/10.1177/016502548901200102

Ryff, C. D. (1995). Psychological well-being in adult life. *Current Directions in Psychological Science, 4*, 99–104. https://doi.org/10.1111/1467-8721.ep10772395

Ryff, C. D. (2017). Eudaimonic well-being, inequality, and health: recent findings and future directions. *International Review of Economics, 64*, 159–178. https://doi.org/10.1007/s12232-017-0277-4

Ryff, C. D. (2018). Well-being with soul: science in pursuit of human potential. *Perspectives on Psychological Science, 13*, 242–248. https://doi.org/10.1177/1745691617699836

Ryff, C. D., & Keyes, C. L. M. (1995). The structure of psychological well-being revisited. *Journal of Personality and Social Psychology, 69*, 719. https://doi.org/10.1037/0022-3514.69.4.719

Salomon, J. A., Wang, H., Freeman, M. K., Vos, T., Flaxman, A. D., Lopez, A. D., & Murray, C. J. L. (2012). Healthy life expectancy for 187 countries, 1990–2010: a systematic analysis for the Global Burden Disease Study 2010. *The Lancet, 380*, 2144–2162. https://doi.org/10.1016/S0140-6736(12)61690-0

Sameroff, A. (Ed.). (2009). *The transactional model of development: how children and contexts shape each other*. American Psychological Association. https://doi.org/10.1037/11877-000.

Schafer, M. H., Ferraro, K. F., & Mustillo, S. A. (2011). Children of misfortune: early adversity and cumulative inequality in perceived life trajectories. *American Journal of Sociology, 116*, 1053–1091. https://doi.org/10.1086/655760

Schilling, O. (2006). Development of life satisfaction in old age: another view on the "Paradox". *Social Indicators Research, 75*, 241–271. https://doi.org/10.1007/s11205-004-5297-2

Schulz, R., Wahl, H.-W., Matthews, J. T., De Vito Dabbs, A., Beach, S. R., & Czaja, S. J. (2015). Advancing the aging and technology agenda in gerontology. *The Gerontologist, 55*, 724–734. https://doi.org/10.1093/geront/gnu071

Schüz, B., Tesch-Römer, C., & Wurm, S. (2014). District-level primary care supply buffers the negative impact of functional limitations on illness perceptions in older adults with multiple illnesses. *Annals of Behavioral Medicine, 49*, 463–472. https://doi.org/10.1007/s12160-014-9671-2

Sen, A. (1993). Capability and well-being. In M. C. Nussbaum & A. Sen (Eds), *The quality of life* (pp. 30–53). Clarendon.

Settersten, R. A., Jr. (2017). Some things I have learned about aging by studying the life course. *Innovation in Aging, 1*, igx014. https://doi.org/10.1093/geroni/igx014

Sholl, J., & Rattan, S. I. S. (2019). Biomarkers of health and healthy ageing from the outside-in. In A. Moskalev (Ed.), *Biomarkers of human aging*. (pp. 37–46). Springer Nature. https://doi.org/10.1007/978-3-030-24970-0_4

Silva, T. N. (2013). Paterson and Zderad's humanistic theory entering the between through being when called upon. *Nursing Science Quarterly, 26*, 132–135. https://doi.org/0.1177/0894318413477209

Spector, W. D., & Fleishman, J. A. (1998). Combining activities of daily living with instrumental activities of daily living to measure functional disability. *The Journal of Gerontology Series B: Psychological Sciences and Social Sciences, 53B*, S46–S57. https://doi.org/10.1093/geronb/53B.1.S46

Stallard, E. (2016). Compression of morbidity and mortality: new perspectives. *North American Actuarial Journal, 20*, 341–354. https://doi.org/10.1080/10920277.2016.1227269

Staudinger, U. M. (2001). Life reflection: a social–cognitive analysis of life review. *Review of General Psychology, 5*, 148–160. https://doi.org/10.1037/1089-2680.5.2.148

Staudinger, U. M., & Baltes, P. B. (1996). Interactive minds: a facilitative setting for wisdom-related performance? *Journal of Personality and Social Psychology, 71*, 746–762. https://doi.org/10.1037/0022-3514.71.4.746

Staudinger, U. M., Marksiske, M., & Baltes, P. B. (1995). Resilience and reserve capacity in later adulthood: potentials and limits of development across the life span. In D. Cicchetti & D. J. Cohen (Eds), *Developmental psychopathology. Volume 2: Risk, disorder, and adaptation* (pp. 801–847). Wiley.

Steels, S. (2015). Key characteristics of age-friendly cities and communities: a review. *Cities, 47*, 45–52. https://doi.org/10.1016/j.cities.2015.02.004

Stephens, C., & Breheny, M. (2018). *Healthy aging. A capability approach to inclusive policy and practice*. Routledge. https://doi.org/10.4324/9781315639093

Stowe, J. D., & Cooney, T. M. (2015). Examining Rowe and Kahn's concept of successful aging: importance of taking a life course perspective. *The Gerontologist, 55*, 43–50. https://doi.org/10.1093/geront/gnu055

Swift, H. J., Abrams, D., Lamont, R. A., & Drury, L. (2017). The risks of ageism model: how ageism and negative attitudes toward age can be a barrier to active aging. *Social Issues and Policy Review, 11*, 195–231. https://doi.org/10.1111/sipr.12031

Swinkels, J., van Tilburg, T., Verbakel, E., & Broese van Groenou, M. (2019). Explaining the gender gap in the caregiving burden of partner caregivers. *The Journal of Gerontology: Series B, 74*, 309–317. https://doi.org/10.1093/geronb/gbx036

Tesch-Römer, C. (2005). Universal accommodation? Cross-cultural notes on Brandtstädter's developmental theory of action. In W. Greve, K. Rothermund, & D. Wentura (Eds), *The adaptive self: personal continuity and intentional self-development* (pp. 285–297). Hogrefe.

Tesch-Römer, C. (2012). *Active ageing and quality of life in old age.* United Nations Economic Commission for Europe.

Tesch-Römer, C. (2020). Successful Aging 2.0. In D. Gu & M. E. Dupre (Eds), *Encyclopedia of gerontology and population aging.* Springer. https://doi.org/https:// doi.org/10.1007/978-3-319-69892-2_479-1

Tesch-Römer, C., & Huxhold, O. (2019). Social isolation and loneliness in old age. In O. Braddick (Ed.), *Oxford Research Encyclopedia of Psychology.* Oxford University Press. https://doi.org/ 10.1093/acrefore/9780190236557.013.335

Tesch-Römer, C., & von Kondratowitz, H.-J. (2006). Comparative ageing research: a flourishing field in need of theoretical cultivation. *European Journal of Ageing, 3,* 155–167.

Tesch-Römer, C., & Wahl, H.-W. (2017). Toward a more comprehensive concept of successful aging: disability and care needs. *The Journal of Gerontology Series B: Psychological Sciences and Social Sciences, 72,* 310–318. https://doi.org/10.1093/ geronb/gbw162

Tesch-Römer, C., & Wurm, S. (2012). Research on active aging in Germany. *GeroPsych, 25,* 167–170. https://doi.org/10.1024/1662-9647/a000067

Tesch-Römer, C., Motel-Klingebiel, A., & Tomasik, M. J. (2008). Gender differences in subjective well-being: comparing societies with respect to gender equality. *Social Indicators Research, 82,* 329–349. https://doi.org/10.1007/s11205-007-9133-3

Timonen, V. (2016). *Beyond successful aging and active ageing. A theory of model ageing.* Policy Press.

Tornstam, L. (2005). *Gerotranscendence: a developmental theory of positive aging.* Springer Publishing.

Tronto, J. C. (2014). Care ethics. In M. T. Gibbons, D. Coole, E. Ellis, & K. Ferguson (Eds), *The encyclopedia of political thought* (pp. 442–443). Wiley-Blackwell.

UNDP. (2020). *Human Development Report 2020: the next frontier. Human development and the Anthropocene.* United Nations Development Programme.

Vaiserman, A. M. (Ed.). (2019). *Early life origins of ageing and longevity.* Springer Nature. https://doi.org/10.1007/978-3-030-24958-8.

Vaiserman, A. M., Lushchak, O. V., & Koliada, A. K. (2016). Anti-aging pharmacology: promises and pitfalls. *Ageing Research Reviews, 31,* 9–35. https://doi.org/ 10.1016/j.arr.2016.08.004

Vaughan, M., LaValley, M. P., AlHeresh, R., & Keysor, J. J. (2016). Which features of the environment impact community participation of older adults? A systematic review and meta-analysis. *Journal of Aging and Health, 28,* 957–978. https://doi.org/ 10.1177/0898264315614008

Vogel, N., Ram, N., Goebel, J., Wagner, G. G., & Gerstorf, D. (2018). How does availability of county-level healthcare services shape terminal decline in well-being? *European Journal of Ageing, 15,* 111–122. https://doi.org/10.1007/ s10433-017-0425-4

Wahl, H.-W. (2016). Life-span developmental psychology and social-behavioral aging science: need for better liaison with life course epidemiology in the future (commentary). *Longitudinal and Life Course Studies*, 7, 174–178. https://doi.org/10.14301/llcs.v7i2.343

Wahl, H.-W. (in press). Three key longings of humankind related to aging seen through the lenses of contemporary gerontology: eternal youth, immortality, and wisdom. In C. Neumann (Ed.), *Old age from antiquity to early modernity: case studies and methodological perspectives*. Neue Reihe der Online-Schriften des DHI Rom.

Wahl, H.-W., & Gerstorf, D. (2018). A conceptual framework for studying COntext Dynamics in Aging (CODA). *Developmental Review*, 50, 155–176. https://doi.org/10.1016/j.dr.2018.09.003

Wahl, H.-W., & Gitlin, L. N. (2018). Linking the socio-physical environment to successful aging: from basic research to intervention to implementation science considerations. In R. Fernández-Ballesteros, A. Benetos, & J.-M. Robine (Eds), *The Cambridge handbook of successful aging* (pp. 570–593). Cambridge University Press. https://doi.org/10.1017/9781316677018.032

Wahl, H.-W., & Weisman, G. D. (2003). Environmental gerontology at the beginning of the new millennium: reflections on its historical, empirical, and theoretical development. *The Gerontologist*, 43, 616–627. https://doi.org/10.1093/geront/43.5.616

Wahl, H.-W., Fänge, A., Oswald, F., Gitlin, L. N., & Iwarsson, S. (2009). The home environment and disability-related outcomes in aging individuals: what is the empirical evidence? *The Gerontologist*, 49, 355–367. https://doi.org/10.1093/geront/gnp056

Wahl, H.-W., Iwarsson, S., & Oswald, F. (2012). Aging well and the environment: toward an integrative model and research agenda for the future. *The Gerontologist*, 52, 306–316. https://doi.org/10.1093/geront/gnr154

Warner, D. F., & Brown, T. H. (2011). Understanding how race/ethnicity and gender define age-trajectories of disability: an intersectionality approach. *Social Science & Medicine*, 72, 1236–1248. https://doi.org/10.1016/j.socscimed.2011.02.034

Webster, J. D. (1993). Construction and validation of the Reminiscence Functions Scale. *Journal of Gerontology*, 48, P256–P262. https://doi.org/10.1093/geronj/48.5.P256

Wettstein, M., Schilling, O. K., Reidick, O., & Wahl, H.-W. (2015). Four-year stability, change, and multidirectionality of well-being in very-old age. *Psychology And Aging*, 30, 500–516. https://doi.org/10.1037/pag0000037

WHO. (2001). *International classification of functioning, disability and health*. World Health Organization.

WHO. (2007). *Global age-friendly cities: a guide*. World Health Organization.

WHO. (2020a). *Decade of healthy ageing 2020–2030*. World Health Organization.

WHO. (2020b). *Decade of healthy ageing: baseline report*. World Health Organization.

Wiener, J. M., Hanley, R. J., Clark, R., & Van Nostrand, J. F. (1990). Measuring the activities of daily living: comparisons across national surveys. *Journal of Gerontology*, 45, S229–S237. https://doi.org/10.1093/geronj/45.6.S229

Wilkinson, L. R., Ferraro, K. F., & Kemp, B. R. (2017). Contextualization of survey data: what do we gain and does it matter? *Research in Human Development, 14*, 234–252. https://doi.org/10.1080/15427609.2017.1340049

Wilkinson, R. G. (1996). *Unhealthy societies: the afflictions of inequality*. Routledge. https://doi.org/10.4324/9780203421680

Wilson-Genderson, M., & Pruchno, R. (2013). Effects of neighborhood violence and perceptions of neighborhood safety on depressive symptoms of older adults. *Social Science & Medicine, 85*, 43–49. https://doi.org/10.1016/j.socscimed.2013.02.028.

Wong, P. T. P. (1989). Personal meaning and successful aging. *Canadian Psychology/ Psychologie Canadienne, 30*, 516–525. https://doi.org/10.1037/h0079829

Wurm, S., & Tesch-Römer, C. (2021). Late-life adaptation. In F. Maggino (Ed.), *Encyclopedia of quality of life and well-being research*. Springer Nature. https://doi.org/10.1007/978-3-319-69909-7_1608-2

Yates, F. E. (1994). Order and complexity in dynamical systems: homeodynamics as a generalized mechanics in biology. *Mathematical and Computer Modelling, 19*, 49–74. https://doi.org/10.1016/0895-7177(94)90189-9

Zaidi, A., Gasior, K., Zolyomi, E., Schmidt, A., Rodrigues, R., & Marin, B. (2017). Measuring active and healthy ageing in Europe. *Journal of European Social Policy, 27*, 138–157. https://doi.org/10.1177/0958928716676550

Index